RAW KIDS

Transitioning Children to a Raw Food Diet

Revised Edition

Cheryl Stoycoff

D1282501

Living Spirit Press
Books for an Awakening Consciousness

Raw Kids
Transitioning Children to a Raw Food Diet - Revised Edition
Cheryl Stoycoff

ISBN: 978-0-9677852-7-1
4rd Printing of Revised Edition

The information provided in this book is the result of the author's experiences as she transitioned her children to a raw and living food diet. It is not intended to substitute as medical advice and therefore, the author and publisher cannot accept responsibility should any problems arise. Readers should use their own judgement, consult a holistic medical expert or their child's pediatrician for specific applications to individual problems.

Published by

 Living Spirit Press
Books for an Awakening Consciousness

P. O. Box 924, Claremore, OK 74018
Email: info@livingspiritfoundation.org
www.livingspiritfoundation.org

Printed in the United States by Morris Publishing
3212 East Highway 30
Kearney, NE 68847
1-800-650-7888

For Zack and Kyle

Author's Note: For ease in communication, your child's gender is referred to as male throughout this book. This liberty has been taken to avoid the awkward use of he/she or him/her.

Also by Cheryl Stoycoff

Soul Speak: Opening to Divine Guidance

Published under Cheryl's new name, Solomae Sananda

The Narrow Path: Revelations in Advanced Spirituality

Kundalini and the Evolution of Consciousness

The Wisdom of Solomae

Ascension Through the Chakras:
The Human Experience of Conscious Evolution

Table of Contents

Prologue to Revised Edition

This is the first revision to *Raw Kids*, which was first published five years ago. Much has changed since our initial experience with raw foods. We have founded a non-profit spiritual organization (The Living Spirit Foundation) and moved from California to the mid-west. I have legally changed my name to Solomae Sananda and under that name; I have written and published four more books. My sons, Zack and Kyle are now sixteen and thirteen respectively. They are an active part of our ministry and also work to educate their peers with regard to a healthy diet and lifestyle.

In this revised addition, I have added two chapters; Cautions and Concerns and Intuitive Eating as well as interspersing some of our experiences gained through the past five years. I felt it important to include a chapter on Cautions and Concerns because of our own experience with the raw food movement and my contact with many parents who faced difficult challenges and problems with the raw food diet for their children. In the chapter entitled Intuitive Eating, I have shared a more in-depth description of my own raw food journey and how that has evolved to this point. I have included this chapter due to the many inquiries I have received over the years. The importance of keeping perspective and finding balance cannot be overstated. In learning to listen to your body, rather than following some externally created ideal, you will be better able to continue growing into greater health and wellness.

May your life be filled with joy and peace and may you know the Presence of God in each moment.

Solomae Sananda, Dec., 2004

i

Introduction

There are many reasons we, as parents, aspire to improve our children's diets. Some are searching for relief from behavioral disorders, some are trying to alleviate a specific health issue, some are trying to avoid a food allergen and others are just trying to improve their children's health in general. No matter what reason you cite, your underlying motivation is the love you have for your child and the responsibility you feel to do what's best for him.

This book is written with the assumption that you already understand the benefits of a raw and living food diet and that you have educated yourself with regard to incorporating this change into your life. That's the easy part. Changing your diet is one thing, but changing the diet of your child, especially when they are too young to understand the reasons, is quite another. There are many different issues that come into play when we try to implement a change in diet for our children. They may not like the change, your relatives or spouse may not understand, there are social pressures, school lunches, holidays, and your own self doubts and insecurities to deal with. Worst of all, there is very little support or information available from the usual sources (pediatricians, nutritionists, etc.).

Even though my husband, Clyde, and I had been following a raw food diet, we were reluctant to make this change for our children, Zack (then age 10) and Kyle (then age 7). Our reluctance was not because we weren't convinced of the superior nutrition and appropriateness of this diet but, because the change seemed too daunting a task. To ask a child to stop eating everything they love and to be so different from other children seemed unfair. This changed however, when we discovered Kyle's diet was affecting his behavior and his ability to learn. The following is an article I wrote regarding our raw food journey with Kyle. It appeared in *Living Nutrition Magazine* (volume 6, 1999).

Triumph over Attention Deficient Disorder via the Raw Food Diet!

My son Kyle is a beautiful, bright and energetic seven year old. He laughs a lot, loves life and makes friends easily. However, since he began school, we have been aware of a problem in his learning ability. He did not learn things as easily as his brother had. Everything was difficult. His teachers complained of his short attention span and were frustrated by his inability to stay focused. They usually had him sit close to the front of the class so they could "keep an eye on him."

In kindergarten, then in first grade, we heard the same thing. The teachers would say Kyle was falling behind the other children. His reading and math were below grade level. His teachers gave him special tutoring and we supplemented that with extra help at home on a daily basis. The problem wasn't bad enough to be called "learning disabled," but the term "Attention Deficient Disorder" (ADD) had been thrown around.

We were adamantly opposed to any type of medication (drug) to alter his behavior and we kept searching for a solution,all the while hoping we could just get him through school.

We knew our son and we knew there was something that was keeping him from grasping what he was being taught. It was as though there was a fog around his brain; the information would go in but he was unable to comprehend or retain it. We witnessed his frustration as he tried so hard to remember and to do what was expected of him. His behavior at home was erratic at times, with frequent quarreling with his brother and periods of extreme moodiness.

Because I had been studying holistic nutrition and natural hygiene and had recently changed to a raw food diet myself, I wondered if Kyle's behavior could be related to something he was eating. He was already eating a "relatively healthy" diet (or so I thought) by society's standards. He was vegan (no animal products), ate no refined sugar, white flour products, junk or processed foods. However, Kyle usually ate wheat at every meal, in some form or another. I knew wheat was a common allergen, so we decided to eliminate wheat from his diet and see if there would be any change. Within days of eliminating wheat the change was incredible! He was calmer, happier and began bringing home 100's on his spelling tests. His teacher called and said she was moving Kyle into one of her "higher groups" as he was doing so well! This was all within 10 days of eliminating wheat from his diet!

This improvement continued for a couple of months but then began to decline. His reading and math were not improving and he was still below grade level. His teacher warned us he would have to be retained, rather than pass to the third grade. His behavior at home became erratic again, even more so than before. At this point, I consulted Dave Klein, whom I had met through the Living and Raw Foods Internet site. I explained Kyle's situation and Dave advised there was still too much starch in Kyle's diet and it was probably fermenting and affecting his brain chemistry. As I evaluated his diet, I realized the wheat had been filled in with vegetables and wheat alternatives (corn tortillas, rice cereals, rice pasta, potatoes and tofu); I had mainly substituted one cooked starch for another! His problem wasn't with wheat—it was with cooked starch! I immediately eliminated the cooked starch and replaced it with vegetables and high fat plant foods and the change was again, immediate. The following is a letter I sent to Dave to update him on Kyle's progress:

"Dear Dave: Just wanted to give you an update on my son, Kyle. Thank you again for your advice—it did the trick! Three weeks ago we took him off cooked starch (cold turnip!) He has been all raw ever since, except for a baked yam or potato once a week. The difference was drastic and immediate! Within three days, his temperament calmed down and he began acting more mature and focused. He even speaks differently, more maturely (slowly and calmly). After about six days, he had some detox—he stayed home from school and for two days complained that"he felt bad all over." (I remember that feeling from my own detox.) This episode was followed by four or five days of intense sleep, then he seemed to bounce back and now feels wonderful! The clincher is this: About six weeks ago I had a parent-teacher conference with his second grade teacher. (I had told you before that he was "slow" and had trouble focusing in school, since Kindergarten). Anyway, six weeks ago the teacher told me that he was reading below grade level and she was going to have to retain him, instead of passing him to third grade. He was required to read at a level sixteen and at that time he was only at a level six. She didn't want us to be shocked when June rolled around and wanted to prepare us. Today, we had another parent-teacher conference. The teacher was so surprised by his "turn around" she had to tell us. She tested him this week and he is now reading at a level ten! She said this rapid of a turnaround is unheard of. She said Kyle is trying so hard and is progressing so fast "all of a sudden" that she is recommending he be moved to third grade, even if he is not quite at a level sixteen by June. (We had told her about his "food-allergies" and that the change in his diet is what we attributed his turnaround to, but she seemed oblivious to the diet/behavior connection.) Now that his brain is working clearly, we have no doubt he will be caught up with his classmates in no time. This is so wonderful! Thank you again for your help!"

About a week after our last conference, Kyle's teacher called to tell us she tested Kyle again on his reading and moved him up to a level twelve. It is truly incredible to see how quickly he is improving now that his brain can function normally. I feel as though some incredible secret has been revealed (it has!). I am overwhelmed when I think of all we have been through in the past two years trying to help him and I am so thankful to have found the most natural and simplest of answers; the raw food diet.

Kyle understands the reason things are easier for him now is because he has changed his diet and he has taken to it like a trooper. Sometimes, there are "challenges," especially in social situations, but having him function and live life to his full potential is worth any bit of awkwardness or inconvenience that being on a different diet may bring.

Since that article appeared, I have been in contact with many parents who are searching for help in the day-to-day transition for their own children. It is apparent to me that there is a need for this type of information. When we began Kyle's transition, I searched for help and although I found many sources of information and advice, none was directed at children. Most of the sources I found did not have children of their own and the parents who were raising their children in the raw food lifestyle had been feeding them this way since birth. In the beginning, there were many trials and errors as we found what worked for us. In this book, I have taken you "between the lines" of our transition. Even though we experienced amazing results, the road was not always smooth. As Kyle has grown, he has changed, and out of necessity, so did my approach and methods. I hope my experience can help smooth the way for all who aspire to pass on the gift of radiant health to their children.

Please note: The inclusion of more fresh fruits and vegetables and the exclusion of animal products and processed foods is such an improvement over the diet of most children in our society, that even implementing these changes can be difficult for some. In transitioning our children, we are teaching them how to care for their bodies for a lifetime. Because they are children, the psychological aspects of diet cannot be ignored. The way in which we approach the change and the way they feel about it determines if they will rebel or embrace this health supporting diet as they grow older. To make a peaceful and lasting change, it is important to start from whatever point you're at. For that reason, I have included some transition tips which include cooked food alternatives to the previously followed diet. It is my opinion that even though the inclusion of these cooked foods is "less harmful" than the Standard American Diet (SAD), they should be used as transition foods and gradually reduced or eliminated in the diet.

In my experience, it can be difficult to strictly follow proper food combining principles when transitioning children away from a cooked and processed diet. For this reason, I have taken liberty with these principles in an attempt to eliminate the harmful foods and incorporate only whole, natural, unfired foods as the sole diet for my children. The guidelines and meal suggestions presented in this book are the result of my experience as I transitioned my own children to a raw and living food diet and are not presented as nutritional recommendations or medical advice.

Chapter 1
You are the Key

The level of success you have in improving your child's diet depends on you. You will need to arm yourself with the nutritional facts, brace yourself for the opposition and use your ingenuity and creativity as never before. You will need undying persistence and confidence that what you are doing is best for your child. Above all, you will need patience with your child and yourself as you experiment and learn together. This is a whole new world, you are trying to change something that has been ingrained since birth (for you and your child).

Your child will look to you as an example. If you are still indulging in that morning cup of coffee and donut or slipping in a candy bar when you think no one is looking, you will not fool your child. Your actions speak much louder than your words. Children are intuitive, inquisitive and smart. We don't give them enough credit. If you are feeling ambivalent about making healthy changes in your own diet, how can you expect your child to embrace these changes? They will sense it if you are explaining something to them and don't really believe it. Your confidence and resolve are imperative. Understand however, that any transition is an ongoing learning experience and above all, one should keep their sense of humor and remain flexible.

1

Even when we are sure we are on the right track with our own dietary transition and we directly experience the benefits of a raw food diet, we are still cautious when it comes to our children. This is understandable. We are willing to experiment with our own health but, naturally are more protective and hesitant in making changes for our children. The change in Kyle's diet brought up some issues for me as a mother. Eventually, I embraced them as an opportunity to further let go of the paradigms that I found were more heavily entrenched with regard to my children. But, early on, certain situations caused doubts to creep in. For example, Kyle spent the night with a friend one evening and I immediately was worried about what he would eat. When the mother came to pick him up, she asked what he could eat. (We had previously told her he was allergic to wheat.) She said she was serving cheese quesadilla for dinner (flour tortillas with cheese melted inside). I told her he was not to have any wheat or animal products. She asked what he could eat and I told her; fruit, vegetables or nuts. Hearing these words come out of my mouth, telling another mother what my son was allowed to eat was very sobering to me. It sounded like I was drastically restricting the options available to my child. There is a double standard at work here. The diet that we follow for ourselves, even after much research and direct experience, is put to further scrutiny when we impose it on our children. This is especially so when we go against what so many people perceive is the "right" and "normal" way to eat.

After that experience, to counter the self doubts that set in, I began pouring over nutritional information verifying what I already knew; that a diet of fresh fruit, vegetables, nuts and seeds provides everything his body needs to be healthy, and *none* of the things that contribute to disease and imbalance. The tables listing the protein content of foods, the amino acid complement found in nuts and the vitamin and mineral content of fruits and vegetables provided the evidence I needed; scientific facts telling me this diet is nutritionally sound.

However, the issue I was dealing with was not an issue of logic or science. It was an issue of societal conditioning. I asked myself if the reason I was uneasy was because of what people may think or say about how I raise my children. There was no doubt that I was going against what the masses viewed as "normal" and acceptable. Our ideas, beliefs and actions are a result of our expanded awareness and willingness to trust our inner guidance, rather than follow what society has placed before us as the "correct" way to live. This is a foreign concept to most of society and I had to find peace and confidence in what I was doing.

To say that our children eat a "vegan diet consisting of predominately fresh fruits and vegetables in their natural state" should not pose a problem. If we succumb to the pressures of society and allow them to eat unhealthy foods because "everyone else does"or alter the way we believe to "fit in" with the mainstream, how will things ever change? If we don't stand up and live our truth, how will the world ever change? It's up to the people who have expanded and awakened to present an example for others who are trying to "go against the crowd." This may be viewed as radical, to be sure it will be viewed as extreme, but no matter. Nothing was ever changed through moderate measures. Half-truths and compromises do not change things, they only allow the "flow" to continue as it has been.

Our children are the benefactors of our expanded awareness. What good does it do for us to obtain higher awareness and knowledge if we don't pass it on to our children? The evolution of expansion must continue onward, generation after generation. Further, this teaches them that it's ok to be different, to follow their own truth, to listen to their body and to nature, rather than follow the masses. This teaches them to question what is presented to them and to think and feel for themselves.

The rationale that doubts if the raw-food diet is healthy for children is the same as saying that adults need to cut back on cholesterol and fat to reduce their risk of heart disease, but it is ok for children to continue to indulge in cheeseburgers because they are not yet "at risk" for heart disease. It's just common sense that if nature has provided foods to nourish our adult bodies, that these same foods provide all that children need as well.

When you consider this point, it is probably even more important for children to eat in a natural, healthy way because from the moment of birth they are growing the bones, teeth, tissues, etc. that will serve them the rest of their lives. Like a house built with a substandard foundation, children who grow their bodies without the optimal foundation, will find their "house" weak and unable to serve them for a lifetime, as it was intended.

The conflict I experienced is a good example of how the ingrained patterns, (the mass consciousness that we are all exposed to since birth) can override and cloud our judgements. The urge to "fit in" and to be viewed as a "good mother" is strong. Everyone takes an overprotective stance on behalf of children because they are unable to choose for themselves. As parents we are held to higher standards as the guardians of these special little people who look to us to show them the way. Naturally, we want the best for our children and we don't want them to suffer for our mistakes or misjudgements, so perhaps, it's correct that we feel this double standard toward our offspring. Nonetheless, it is important to realize that conformity for the sake of appearance helps no one. Instead, the concern and action should be the education of yourself with facts to substantiate your beliefs, the firm conviction (based on your inner knowing) that the way you are living is in alignment with nature and, above all, the right motivation (love) for your course of action. When these are present, there is no need for defensiveness. There is only the light that shines from within, outward to illuminate the world. Your child can't help but flourish in this light.

foods as motivation. Her son enjoyed the increased endurance and ability to run farther and faster than he did before. He liked the lightness he experienced just after eating and complained about the feeling of heaviness after eating a cooked meal. This boy was only eight, but that's old enough to recognize what feels good in his body and what doesn't.

Sometimes a child may have a physical problem, such as constipation, rashes, allergies, asthma, etc. that can be alleviated with a raw food diet. These are profound motivators for experimenting with a change in diet. The possibility of giving up medications and being able to participate in life as other children, can make even the reluctant child try something new.

This "immediate payoff" is important for children because they are unable to see things in the long term. There needs to be something tangible they can derive from improving their diets in order to make them a willing participant. Get imaginative here. Maybe they are tired of helping clean the kitchen and doing the dishes. Point out that raw foods require little preparation and therefore, little clean up. Make them a fruit smoothie or frozen sorbet and tell them they get to eat dessert for lunch! It's important that you have made up your mind and are confident in your decision. When you discuss these changes with your child, present it in a way that says, "this is what we are going to do." There is no room for ambiguity. Let them know these changes *are going to happen* and then proceed to discuss the why and how of them.

You must speak to your children as the people they are. They are capable of understanding much more than we give them credit for. Speak to them about the earth and the environment. Show them the difference in packaging and garbage when we eat food in it's natural state compared to the packaged convenience foods most people eat. Talk to them about pollution and explain how a diet of animal products depletes the earth's resources. Plant a tree with them. Grow a garden. Grow sprouts and greens for your salads. Teach them to feed themselves. Who knows what the world will be like when they are adults. They may need these basic forgotten skills just to survive.

I remember a conversation we had over the dinner table six years ago. Zack, my oldest was five and Kyle was two. We were eating hamburgers (this was before we were vegetarian) and Zack looked at his plate and asked me how they make hamburger. I was startled by his question and I carefully explained that it was made from cows. He looked shocked and quite upset. With wide eyes he looked at me in disbelief and said, "We are eating a dead cow?" (Out of the mouths of babes!) The tone in his voice and his innocence made me question the necessity of eating animals. I remember feeling uncomfortable explaining to my son that hamburgers were made from cows and I realized something was wrong if I felt I had to "soften" the reality of our diet to my five yearold. That experience was the turning point that started my research into vegetarianism. Two months later, I read *Diet for a New America* by John Robbins and our family became vegetarian overnight.

On a more recent occasion, Kyle had played in a soccer game and received a drink and snack after the game. As is our custom, he gave them to me to read the ingredients. I OK'd the juice as it was 100% juice, but the snack was another matter. They were cookies with M & M's in them and as I read the ingredients out loud to Kyle we were both surprised to read "canuba wax" amongst the usual preservatives and food dyes. Kyle stopped me as I read and asked, "What is canuba wax?" I told him it was something they use to wax cars. He was appalled and wanted to know why on earth they would put something that you wax cars with into something you are supposed to eat! This launched a long discussion about the importance of knowing what goes into our bodies.

You need to watch your child's attitude with regard to his diet. You don't want him to feel deprived, like he is being punished or missing out on something. This is a fine line, especially in the early stages of transition. Do not use food as a "treat." If you allow your child to eat something unhealthy on occasion (cake, pizza, ice cream), be careful not to label it a treat. If you do, he will perceive that these things are good, like rewards or special foods that are to be looked forward to. If you do choose to allow him to eat these things, talk about it before hand. Explain that you don't usually eat these things because they are not good for your body but he can have them occasionally if he chooses to. Do not imply that he is "bad" if he chooses to, keep it light, don't place undue importance on one meal. It is also good to talk about how he feels after he eats these foods. The body of a child who has been on a pure foods diet will react adversely when impure foods are eaten. This experience is necessary for him

10

to understand the workings of his body. It may be necessary over and over as he grows. Let him discover this for himself. This direct experience will teach him much more than your words ever could. We don't bring these unhealthy foods into our home but, if my children encounter them in a social situation, they are free to eat them. Since they don't have access to them on a regular basis, there isn't a temptation or feeling of depravation. Out of sight, out of mind.

It's important not to be too ridged in the beginning. You don't want to make the transition to a healthier diet a source of contention in your family. The amount of rigidity will vary depending on your reasons and motivation for implementing the changes. Begin slowly, replacing all snacks with fruit. Then replace one meal a day with salad and baked potato. Serve a smoothie for breakfast instead of cereal or toast. Keep expanding your options. Don't take the mind set that "he won't eat that." NEVER decide ahead of time what your child will eat. This closes all possibilities and brings an element of negativity into your interactions with him. Simply offer him new things, without expectations and let him try them. Don't make him feel he has to eat something, which will only serve to push him in the opposite direction. In our home, we have only one rule; you have to try all mom's new recipes. If you don't try it, how will you know if you like it or not? One bite is all I ask!

There are children who refuse to eat anything but their favorite, unhealthy foods. We have had a couple of episodes of this type with our boys too. We provide healthy, natural, delicious food for them to eat. If they are hungry, they will eat. A child will not starve themselves. It takes fortitude, but you must be lovingly firm. If your child wanted to drink a fifth of vodka, would you give it to him? Of course not, you know it's harmful to him. It's the same with unhealthy foods. Why give your child candy, pastries or hot dogs when you know they are not good for him? Does it matter that the damage takes years to manifest? You may have allowed them to eat these unhealthy foods before, but now that you know better you must follow that truth. You cannot go against what your inner knowing tells you, without eventually suffering the consequences.

What if your child has no interest in improving his diet? This is more likely if the child has been eating the Standard American Diet (SAD), full of processed and fast foods, meat, dairy, sugar and preservatives. In this case, you must trust yourself even more. It's up to you as the parent to do what you feel is best for him. Present your case to him and explain the reasons you are now choosing to eat this way. Share the information you have learned. Allow him to keep the foods that you feel are "less harmful," such as baked potatoes or yams, steamed vegetables, tofu, sprouted wheat bread, steamed brown rice, etc. Provide vegetarian substitutes for animal products. There are vegetarian hot dogs, hamburgers, lunch meats, corn dogs, soy cheeses, rice and soy milk, etc. There is absolutely no reason to continue eating animal products given such a wide and readily available variety of vegetarian substitutes. Once these improvements are made and he is comfortable with them, you can work on transitioning him away from these things. Even if you go no further, this is still a wonderful improvement over what most children eat!

No two children are alike and no two households are alike. You need to start where you are, move forward and never look back. Take each day one at a time, learn from each situation. Treat your child with love and respect and above all, be honest with him. If you do this, you will only know success.

Chapter 3
The Outside World

You're on the right track. You've dealt with your own doubts, you've managed to gain the cooperation of your child, you feel comfortable with your meal choices and daily food plan but, what happens when you have to venture outside?

When we first became vegetarian six years ago, I remember feeling uneasy in social situations (restaurants, holidays, parties, etc.) as we tried to find "something we could eat." I laugh when I look back at this. Being a (cooked food) vegetarian was easy compared to being a raw foodist in those situations. We, as adults, have the ability to explain why we are bringing our own food, carrying that bag into the restaurant, or skipping a meal. For our children, this is another matter. Social situations involving our children do present challenges for those choosing to go against the mainstream. With a little creativity and flexibility, these situations can be managed and even enjoyed.

School Lunches

The issue of school lunches is a big one. We are all aware of the deplorable, nutritional deficient "foods" that are served to our nation's children. For the parent striving to feed their child a pure raw food diet, this issue must be addressed on a daily basis.

15

Since we now home school our children, this is no longer an issue for us but, early in our raw food transition my children still attended public school and I found this to be one of the most challenging areas we encountered. As with everything, you must educate your child. Take the weekly newspaper and read the school lunch menus with your child. Discuss the items served. If you have done your homework, he will already know that hamburgers, hot dogs and pizza are inferior foods and not something you serve in your home. As he faces his school-mates each day, it is important that he have an understanding of why he eats the way he does. Help him to understand that this knowledge he has about the correct way to eat and nourish his body gives him an "edge" over the masses who are overweight, have frequent colds and flu and reduced energy and stamina. Help him understand that as he grows older he won't have to fear the diseases that he has seen around him (cancer, heart disease, diabetes, etc.). Don't impart a feeling of superiority in him, rather, a quiet peace that he is following God's (nature's) plan for his body and the knowledge that as he grows, he can help teach others by his example.

So, what do you send in a raw food sack lunch? We tried everything; celery and carrot sticks with raw almond butter; fruit salad (cut up and ready to eat in a container); raw humus with various vegetables for dipping; blended soups (slightly warmed and kept in a thermos); dehydrated nut/seed crackers; dehydrated cookies; dates; cabbage roll-ups (nut butter, cucumber and sprouts rolled up in a cabbage leaf); carrot-raisin salad; coleslaw. Any fruit can be taken along as it comes in it's own wrapper, all that's required is peeling. If you wish to send banana or apple slices already peeled and cut, simply toss them with a little lemon juice. Avocados are wonderful, I eat one every day, but my children won't touch them. If yours will, you can use avocado to make a spread, dip or guacamole and use that as a base for cabbage roll-ups, as a spread on dehydrated crackers or as a stuffing for hollowed out vegetables. I usually sent a bag of dried fruit and/or nuts with them in addition to their sack lunch. If they were hungry in between, they could munch on these at recess. Dried fruit is a concentrated form of sugar and calories. While adults usually eat dried fruits sparingly due to the density and high concentration of sugar, I find my children thrive having this additional form of calories and glucose in their diets.

If you are not aiming for 100% raw, you can opt for an occasional cafeteria lunch, on the days when they serve a vegetarian option. The menu choices vary from school to school and state to state, but most cafeterias offer bean burritos, grilled cheese sandwiches, meatless chili beans or baked potatoes, occasionally. Many schools now offer salad bars as an option. If you are still providing cooked food choices for your child, you can provide a vegan (no animal products) lunch that is wholesome and a definite improvement over school lunches. Some ideas are; potato, split pea or broccoli soup in a thermos; sandwiches made from sprouted bread, vegetarian lunchmeat and soy cheese; a bean burrito on a whole wheat tortilla; raw nut butter and banana slices. Flexibility is the key. Keep your eyes open for new ideas, don't be confined to the usual brown bag ideas we grew up with. The choices are only as limited as your imagination.

Social Gatherings

Another area of concern that invariably comes up are kid-centered social gatherings. Pizza parties after softball, soccer award dinners, birthday parties and school functions can disrupt your well–laid dietary plans. In the beginning, I fretted to no end about these occasions. I worried Kyle would feel different and I worried the other kids would give him a hard time for not eating as they did. At first, our standard answer was to say Kyle had a "wheat allergy," this alleviated the questions and inquiries.

In avoiding wheat products you are pretty well eliminating the junk food served at these gatherings (cake, cupcakes, cookies, pizza etc.). As time went by and Kyle improved, we relaxed a bit and allowed him a slice of pizza at the end of season team parties and a piece of cake at an annual birthday party. When there has been a gathering that no vegetarian options were available, I would simply take a vegetarian equivalent of whatever was being served. I wish to point out that whenever he did partake in these foods, the entire family noticed the behavioral change in him, which usually lasted about 24 hours. You will have to decide where you draw the line. If your child has a health issue, you may not be able to allow variances from the pure diet. If ths is the case, your child will be aware of the consequences of deviating from his diet and that should make the adherence easier. It's important to keep the issue of diet in perspective. One meal, or even one meal a month is not going to make that much difference in the overall scheme of his life. His health (mental and physical) will be determined by what he does 95% of the time, not the occasional lapse. However, you should be forewarned that the more you allow your child to fluctuate back and forth the harder it will be for him to stick to a pure diet. The body is not able to totally purify if the unhealthy foods continue to circulate through the bloodstream. As the unhealthy substances circulate, cravings result, which leads to a struggle between you and your child. If you recognize this pattern, you may want to reevaluate the frequency in which you make exceptions with his diet.

Restaurant Meals

Restaurant meals are another area in which we must be creative. If you are fortunate enough to live in an area with a vegetarian restaurant, you can usually get a high quality organic salad or other acceptable fruit or vegetable plates. Today, most every restaurant has some vegetarian options on thier menu and most will accommodate a special diet if you ask. If you are not following a 100% raw diet, you can also easily find relatively healthy fare at Mexican restaurants (guacamole tostada without cheese or sour cream); Japanese restaurants (vegetable sushi, cabbage slaw or cucumber salads); or Chinese restaurants (vegetable stir fry dishes). Steamed vegetable or fruit plates are also widely available. When traveling and in doubt, always bring your food. If you have healthy options available for the kids (and you) when hunger strikes, you will be less likely to revert to the familiar (unhealthy) stand-by's to pacify them.

Relatives

The last "outside" issue I wish to address is that of relatives. (I can almost hear you groan in unison as you read that line!) Well–meaning grandparents, aunts and uncles, even spouses can be a source of conflict when they voice their disagreement with the dietary choices you have made for your child. Their disapproval can put us on the defensive and cause family gatherings to be strained and uncomfortable. We have experienced this in our own family. We have relatives who believe a vegetarian diet is unhealthy for children, be it cooked or raw. No amount of factual information, expert opinions, scientific studies or direct observation have been able to convince them otherwise. What is even more frustrating is these types of people usually have no tangible basis for their objections, therefore, there is no platform for debate or discussion.

If you are experiencing a conflict with your relatives regarding your child's diet and you feel the need to rectify the situation, you need to directly address the problem. First, understand they truly have your child's best interest at heart. Their motivation is the same as yours; love for your child. From this understanding, you can proceed to explain why you have chosen to make these changes in diet. Arm yourself with the literature and sources you have accumulated and present your case. Open your mind to their point of view and they will be more open to seeing yours. Understand that they are operating under the same conditioning most of our society is: that we need meat and milk to be healthy. This has been drilled into them since childhood and it is further perpetuated with every commercial and advertisement they see.

Unless they have had a reason to seek out new information, they have had no reason to question these beliefs. Use the opportunity to enlighten them about their own health and nutritional habits. If, after your best attempts, you are unable to enlist their support, you will have to accept this difference of opinion.

Don't let their comments and disapproving attitude affect you. If you do, you will be allowing an element of negativity into your life (specifically surrounding your family's diet) that needn't be there. The raw food diet is about being in balance with nature. It is about operating from an awareness of peace and experiencing that peace within your body. The opinions of those who have yet to achieve this awareness should not disturb this peace.

If the opposition comes from a grandparent, it's easier to dismiss their disapproval because they don't have direct influence over your child. But, if the conflict is arising from the disapproval of the other parent, the situation can be more difficult. I had the opportunity to speak to a father who was trying to transition his son to a raw food diet. When we spoke, he was still transitioning him away from meat and dairy and was trying to get him away from cooked starches, mainly breads and pastas. His wife (the child's mother) was reluctant to make these changes. She felt he needed to eat meat for protein and did not see the harm in his eating some form of bread at every meal. The small changes she did allow were not enough to allow their son's body to cleanse, so they never observed a dramatic improvement in his behavior or relief from his chronic constipation.

The father was understandably frustrated. In this type of situation, when the dietary change is not entirely under your control, you need to do what you can and accept what you cannot change. As with grandparents, you must educate the other parent by sharing the information you have gathered. You need to realize that often, opposition is actually defensiveness stemming from reluctance to change one's own diet.

To agree to a change in diet for your child, you must first look at your own diet. Being hypocritical is not a comfortable place to be. Patience and nonjudgmental sharing of information are the keys.

Sometimes, you can convince the opposing parent to agree to try the new diet for two weeks. Even if they feel a raw vegetarian diet is lacking, they will probably concede that not much damage can be done in two weeks time. At the end of the two week experiment, the three of you (both parents and the child) sit down and reevaluate the situation. Discuss the changes you noticed. Be sure to note everything; health problems that may have improved; your child's attitude; his behavior; ability to communicate and get along with other family members; the difference in your household grocery bill; garbage consumption and general interaction as a family. The raw food diet goes well beyond the physical body. It changes us at an energetic and cellular level. There are many things that are intangible and unmeasurable, but profound nonetheless. This experiment may be all it takes to win them over.

As each of these situations arose, we explored our options and remained open to all possibilities. If we found a conflict arising, we "nipped it in the bud" before it was blown out of proportion. There is nothing that can't be worked out once you have made up your mind to make living and raw foods part of your life. As time goes by, the things that seemed difficult at first, become easy. It's all a matter of perception.

Chapter 4
Nutritional Issues

The first thought that crosses our minds when we look to change our children's diets is their health. We don't want to inadvertently cause them nutritional harm, so we proceed with caution. The nutritional needs of children do differ from adults and therefore, our concern is appropriate. If you are hesitant about committing to this transition fully or, if there is conflict within your family regarding the implementation of these dietary changes, it most probably stems from concern over these differing nutritional needs. Just what do children need? In this chapter, I will attempt to shed some light on this subject.

I would like to point out that although I have studied conventional and holistic nutrition, I am not a registered dietitian. This, I believe is to my credit. Had I been indoctrinated with conventional dogmas regarding the "four food groups," I would not have been open to learning from my own experience and observation.

The idea that we need charts and guidelines to tell us how much of what foods we need to eat each day is absurd. Do we really believe mankind was doomed to malnutrition before science isolated and named a few nutritional components?

When we trust in nature and allow our bodies to lead us, there is no need for scientific interference. If I eat a lot of sweet fruit (dates, bananas, etc.) my body tells me I need to eat green salad. When I eat a lot of salad, my body craves avocados and nuts. In this way, our bodies maintain balance. Our children are no different. As I changed my boy's diets, I took my ques from them. Some days they want nuts all day. Other days, they are happy with fruit. I try to follow proper food combining guidelines but most importantly, I follow them. When you think about it, would our bodies be created without the inherent knowledge they need to thrive? Does any other animal on the planet need instructions to tell it what it needs to eat? It's due to man's interference with our natural food supply that we have been cut off from the awareness of this guidance and the faith it takes to listen to it. Something so natural and basic should not be complicated and confusing.

I know everyone is not as trusting as I, and if you are trying to convince a reluctant spouse, relative or pediatrician, you need something more concrete to present your case. Those who need reassurance from "experts" will be pleased to read the following excerpts from the American Dietetic Association's position paper on vegetarian diets[1]:

"It is the position of the American Dietetic Association that appropriately planned vegetarian diets are healthful, are nutritionally adequate, and provide health benefits in the prevention and treatment of certain diseases."

"Well–planned vegan and lacto–ovo–vegetarian diets are appropriate for all stages of the life cycle, including during pregnancy and lactation. Appropriately planned vegan and lacto–ovo–vegetarian diets satisfy nutrient needs of infants, children, and adolescents and promote normal growth."

The following guidelines are then added:

"Choose a variety of foods, including whole grains, vegetables, fruits, legumes, nuts, seeds and, if desired, dairy products and eggs."

"Choose whole, unrefined foods often and minimize intake of highly sweetened, fatty, and heavily refined foods"

"Do not restrict fat in children younger than two years. For older children, include some foods higher in unsaturated fats (e.g., nuts, seeds, nut and seed butters, avocado, and vegetable oils) to help meet energy needs."

In reading the above, it's clear that even the American Dietetic Association has given a green light to a vegan diet for children. The issue as to whether these vegan foods (fruits, vegetables, nuts, seeds and grains) need to be cooked is not addressed. However, I don't think anyone would argue the point that there is more nutritional value in uncooked foods than in cooked. The vitamin, mineral and enzyme loss in cooked foods is well documented. The question to ask yourself (and anyone you are trying to convince) is, "What is it cooked foods provide that the same food in it's raw state can't?" Once you acknowledge that a plant–based diet provides everything the body needs and there is no nutritional benefit (only nutritional detriment) in cooking these plant foods, the argument against a raw food diet disappears. Because they are still growing and are more physically active, children have a need for more calories and fat in their diets than do adults. These needs are easy to satisfy simply by following the body's signals. When my boys are expending a lot of energy, they are hungrier. They eat until they are satiated. They eat as often as they need, listening to their body's signals, rather than following some structured meal time plan.

In my kitchen, I have baskets of fresh fruit (bananas, apples, oranges, grapefruit, persimmons, kiwi, etc.) In our pantry are jars of raw almonds, walnuts, macadamias, filberts, sunflower and pumpkin seeds, dried apricots, pineapple and apple. In the refrigerator we have dates, manna bread[2], carrot and celery sticks, melons and raw nut butters. On our windowsill are jars of sprouts (alfalfa, lentil, mung bean, buckwheat and sunflower). When I prepare food for my boys, I always think of ways to add fat and calories. Neither one likes avocados, so I use other plant fats. When I make a smoothie, I include nut milk or a couple tablespoons of raw sesame tahini. In our salad dressings we use cold–pressed olive oil and sunflower or pumpkin seeds for a base. We also include several olives with each salad. In the winter, there is an increased need for fat as the body adjusts itself to the colder temperatures. I have noticed during this time they naturally eat more nuts and dried fruit. In the spring, as the weather changes, they gravitate toward more fresh fruit.

Juicing is another way to quell your fears about your child getting enough nutrients. When we began the boys on raw foods, we introduced them to carrot juice. It was *not* a big hit. So, I tried making the juice 50% apple and 50% carrot. This went over well, and I gradually reduced the apple until it is now 90% carrot and 10% apple. In addition, I usually add some kale or spinach in with the carrot, it doesn't take much and this doesn't change the appearance or taste of the juice too much. In the winter, we alternate between our usual carrot juice and fresh squeezed orange or grapefruit juice, taking advantage of the wonderful crop of ripe citrus that's available.

Something I noticed with my boys in the early stages of transition was increased hunger. Like us, they are used to that "full" feeling created by the ingestion of cooked starches and the slow digestion of these substances. Don't assume they are "always hungry" because they are not getting the nutrients they need. It takes time to get used to the lighter, cleaner feeling that comes with eating raw foods. This only lasted a short time before their bodies adjusted and they settled into a rhythm. Like all children, they experience days of increased hunger, usually due to a growth spurt. These days are usually followed by several days of decreased appetite, another example of the body knowing what it needs.

When a child regularly eats processed foods, their taste buds become corrupted by the unnatural sweeteners and increased sodium. The body's signals of hunger and satiation are corrupted as blood sugar levels fluctuate and the senses are dulled, resulting in cravings and binges on these unnatural foods. The body's natural rhythm is thrown off in an attempt to assimilate all that it is ingesting. The organism adapts as best it can. As the body is allowed to purify, the taste buds are "reset" and balance restored. Early into our transition, I was happy to find my boys asking for fresh foods and enjoying salads they previously didn't care for. Once the unnatural foods were out of their diets, their natural instincts took over.

Grains

There are differing opinions among raw foodist as to whether we should consume grains at all. During Kyle's initial cleansing period, we did cut out all grain products but have since added in moderate amounts of sprouted, uncooked grains. For example, we use Essene bread made from sprouted wheat and Kyle enjoys a breakfast cereal of sprouted buckwheat and raisins (see recipe section). I have found these additions a helpful inclusion in the boys' diet as they add caloric density and essential amino acids. In addition, because they are sprouted, they are a living food. Since the addition of these sprouted grains, we have not seen any recurrence of Kyle's previous difficulties.

Raw Milk

Since the first publication of Raw Kids, we have made a wonderful discovery...raw milk! Having none of the detriments which occur through the pasteurization and homogenization process, raw milk provides calcium, protein, vitamin

D and is soothing to the nervous system, providing the necessary amino acids and fats for nerve conductivity. Raw organic milk, from a good and natural source is pure prana. It is life-giving and life-sustaining. I have heard many raw-food vegans say that over the long term, they were able to sustain their raw diet through the inclusion of raw dairy products. We are fortunate enough to have a dairy close to our home that sells raw, organic milk directly to the public. In some states, you can find it in natural food stores and co-ops.

What About Protein?

This is by far the most common question asked of vegans (cooked or raw). When we first became vegetarians, I delighted in pointing out to these inquiring minds that we get our protein in the same way the animals they eat get theirs—from plant foods. We're all a product of the advertising campaigns supplied by the meat and dairy industries that have been presented to us as nutritional fact since we were in grade school. We were taught that the only place you can get protein is from animal products. This protein myth dies hard. To change this misconception, we need only look to nature. As babies, we had a higher need for protein than at any other time in our lives. At no other time do our bodies develop and grow at such a rate. What food did nature provide for us as infants? Mother's milk, which is approximately 5% protein. Common sense tells us that as we grow through childhood and later into adulthood, our protein needs would not exceed that of an infant.

Dr. John McDougall states in his book, *The McDougall Program* (Penguin Books, 1990): *"It's extremely hard for anyone to become protein deficient. Unless you gave up eating altogether, I don't see how you'd ever manage it. Virtually all unrefined foods are loaded with proteins. The unfortunate reality is that most Americans consume enormous quantities of unnecessary and excess proteins, which must be excreted through the kidneys, harming them and the rest of the body in the process."*

The World Health Organization sets protein requirements at 4½ percent of caloric intake per day for men, with similar requirements for women and children.[3]

This percentage of protein is not only easy to achieve, it's automatic when eating from the wide range of raw and living foods that are readily available. The following list, from *Nutritive Value of American Foods in Common Units*, U.S.D.A. Agriculture Handbook No. 456, demonstrates the percentage of calories from protein found in raw plant foods:

Vegetables		Fruits		Grains/Nuts/Seeds	
Spinach	49%	Honeydew	16%	Spr. Wheat	18%
Broccoli	45%	Cantaloupe	9%	Buckwheat	15%
Kale	45%	Orange	8%	Walnuts	13%
Lettuce	34%	Apricot	8%	Almonds	12%
Zucchini	28%	Grape	8%	Cashews	12%
Cucumber	24%	Banana	5%	Pumpkin Sds.	21%
Tomato	18%	Apple	1%	Sunflower Sds.	17%

Given this information, protein is clearly not an issue in a raw food diet. I have noticed a pattern with my boys. During periods of growth (growth spurts) they naturally gravitate toward more nuts and nut butters and even request second or third helpings of salad. During these periods of increased protein needs, their bodies naturally tell them what they need. These periods last for a week or two in the spring and again in the fall. Afterwards, they gravitate back to a more balanced intake, increasing fruits and decreasing nuts. This is not something I taught them or a planned dietary regimen they follow. It is simply the natural state of being which emerges when the body is allowed to return to it's natural state.

What About Calories?

Another area of concern regarding children and a raw food diet is that of adequate caloric intake. Does the raw food diet provide enough calories for a growing child? The National Academy of Sciences has set the recommended daily dietary allowances for children as follows:[4]

Ages 1 – 2	900 – 1800 calories
Ages 4 – 6	1300 – 2300 calories
Ages 7 – 10	1650 – 3300 calories

The wide range for each age group is due to variances in height, weight and activity level. Clearly, caloric requirements are an individual issue.

We all know that calories are not created equal. Many children on the SAD (Standard American Diet) consume vast amounts of calories, far exceeding these recommended guidelines. The calories consumed are "empty calories," providing no nutritional value. As a result, they may be receiving enough calories to fill the body's energy needs, but are nutritionally deficient because the calories consumed are not providing the nutrients the body needs to maintain and optimize other functions.

Do you know anyone who calculates and counts the calories they, or their children consume each day? People trying to lose weight may try this approach, but basically, we don't usually worry that we are taking in enough calories because it's such a natural process. It takes care of itself.

The more active your child is, the more calories he needs. To this increased need, his body responds with increased hunger, he eats until his hunger signals cease, naturally satisfying his body's needs. However, this natural bodily response becomes corrupted when we eat unnatural foods. Children who "eat all day" and seemingly cannot get enough food, are experiencing their body's signals for *nutrients*, not calories. When we eat a predominately cooked diet, (especially if it includes refined flour products, sugar and other empty calorie substances) the body doesn't feel satiated because it's hungry for nutrients. When the body signals with hunger, asking for more nutrients, and is given these nutritionally deficient foods, it keeps signaling, demanding what it needs. The result is a body that is overweight (excess calories) but, nutritionally starving. Sadly, this is the state of most of our society today.

Once the body is allowed to purify, and is receiving abundant nutrients from fresh fruits and vegetables, it becomes amazingly efficient at assimilating these nutrients. The results are a decreased appetite and optimized functioning of the body and mind. I am amazed at the decreased amount of food I need now that I am a raw foodist. I can't imagine how I ever managed to eat the typical cooked meals I once did. I have also noticed this in my children. At the beginning of their transition, they were hungrier than they had been before but, after a couple of weeks, their appetites leveled off and adjusted to the higher quality food being consumed. It was as if they needed to pack in the nutrients they had been missing and once their bodies had replenished and stored the nutrients they needed, the increased hunger subsided and they became satiated with less food.

Our bodies, no matter what age they are, come with all they need to maintain health. Within them, our children have all the inherent wisdom they need to grow optimally. It's only in our deviations from what is natural that we cease to understand this and experience the consequences of this deviation.

Let Nature Take it's Course

Being armed with nutritional facts and figures may be helpful to alleviate your doubts and to enlist support from other family members but, it's also important to put those facts and figures into perspective. For me, the beauty of a raw food diet is being able to live as we were intended, without concerns about the "food groups" and "recommended daily allowances" and to be free of worry about illness, deficiencies or dietary supplementation. When we eat a raw and living food diet, the established dietary requirements, guidelines, and charts become meaningless. The causes of disease become apparent and the way to radiant health, obvious. Science may have isolated a few nutrients and even discovered what they do within the body, but we can never hope to fully understand the inherent wisdom and perfect mechanisms at work within our bodies. We need only withdraw our interference and let nature take it's course.

[1]This position paper appeared in the Journal of American Dietetic Association, November 1997, Volume 97, Number 11.

[2]Unleavened bread made from sprouted wheat, also known as Essene bread.

[3]Protein Requirements, Food and Agricultural Organization, World Health Organization Expert Group, United Nations Conference Rome, 1965.

[4]From Recommended Dietary Allowances, 9th ed. National Academy of Sciences, Washington, DC. 1980.

Chapter 5
The Diet–Behavior Connection

Parents don't need scientific studies to tell them the food their child eats affects his behavior. Attend a typical child's birthday party, an hour after cake and punch is served and you can observe it for yourself. Any school teacher will tell you the weeks after Halloween and Easter are two of the worst of the year. Typically, sugar has been the scapegoat, the culprit blamed for the hyperactivity and unruliness. I have discovered, that there are many more subtle and far reaching things that are affected by our children's diet. And, I have been surprised to learn what should have been apparent all along; that when we eat anything that is altered from its natural state, it alters *us* from our natural state. So it is with our children. Perhaps, we don't even know who they really are, having never experienced their company, nor seen their potential expressed through a pure and detoxified body.

To observe the change in my son's behavior as a result of the transition to a raw food diet has been amazing. Just as we saw an immediate, drastic improvement in his behavior when he ate predominately raw and living foods, we likewise saw an immediate recurrence of these undesirable behaviors when he ate cooked or processed foods.

As I explained in the introduction, it was Kyle's symptoms of ADD (Attention Deficit Disorder) and his inability to learn that served as our motivation to change his diet. More recently, we eliminated wheat products from Kyle's diet, thinking he had an allergy to wheat. Although there was an immediate improvement, it soon diminished as the wheat was replaced by other cooked starches.

In observing Kyle it has become obvious which foods affect his behavior. As his body has become more purified, his reactions are more apparent and immediate, providing the perfect situation for experimentation and observation. Initially, we cut out all cooked foods. We call this the "cleansing period." This lasted about two months, even though we were able to see very drastic changes in a matter of days. After the initial two months, we added back in a baked potato or baked yam twice a week. He eats this with his evening salad. This resulted in no difference in behavior, so we occasionally let him have some brown rice and steamed vegetables. So far, this has worked wonderfully. Kyle eats predominately raw foods, with the above items a few nights a week. I have not seen any recurrence in his problem behaviors on this regimen. I do feel it is imperative to have the cleansing period in which no cooked foods are eaten if you are transitioning your child for a specific behavioral or physical problem. This is the only way to allow the body to clean out the offending residue and it provides a clear field for you to assess the improvement.

There have been times when we have allowed Kyle to stray from the raw food plan, usually for social occasions or school functions. During these times, the foods that produce the worst effects are the cooked grain products (breads, cakes, cookies, pizza, etc.) these, together with sugar, are at the top of our "avoid at all costs" list. Basically, a diet of fresh, raw fruit, vegetables, nuts, seeds and sprouted grains, with some occasional cooked vegetables seems optimal, providing the most flexibility, variety and degree of satiety.

The behavior your child exhibits directly influences how others treat him. When a child is not given the chance to experience a pure, optimally functioning physical body, he is not able to relate to those around him in a way that builds strong, loving relationships. Of course, we love our children but, what parent can't relate to the frustration of dealing with a demanding, high-maintenance child on a daily basis? Many times, these children go through their entire childhoods un-aware that what they are eating contributes to or causes their behavioral problems. Unfortunately, these children usually receive a label such as "hyperactive," "difficult" or "slow," which follows them throughout childhood and influences how they view themselves and how others treat them. Often, neither the child nor the parent realizes there is a problem, having grown so used to these behaviors and devising various methods of dealing with them. If others (his teacher, his siblings, his parents) perceive him as a "problem" because of his behavior, that perception is reflected back to the child. It becomes his perception of himself. If he constantly operates in a "fog", unable to grasp fully the world around him, his education suffers, setting him up for future difficulties as he goes through life. That is why it is so important to understand the diet–behavior connection and to understand that what the child eats not only influences his behavior but, how others treat him and therefore, how he views himself and his place in the world.

You know your child as no one else. You know when he is experiencing difficulty or frustration. You know when he is intentionally misbehaving and when he doesn't seem to be able to help himself. Children are a precious joy, their diet should not make them unpleasant to be around or create difficulty in their life. It is up to you to make the changes necessary to allow your child the best chance to grow up happy, healthy and peacefully.

Chapter 6
Spiritual Issues

I would be remiss if I did not include this chapter, given our experience and the changes the raw food lifestyle has brought into our lives. Once your child is allowed to return to a more balanced state of being, all aspects of his life (and yours) will be affected. Since we are not just physical beings, we must understand that the state of our mind and bodies effects every aspect of our lives.

Whatever your reasons for wanting to implement these changes into your child's diet, you should realize that in going against the mainstream in something so basic as the food he eats, you are taking the first steps in "unplugging" him from the craziness of our modern world. The raw food diet soon becomes a lifestyle as you and your child share the experience of growing your own food (sprouting, gardening, etc.), reconnecting with the earth as the source of nourishment and recognizing yourselves as an integral part of the circle of life. These transformations intertwine themselves throughout your lives, changing how you perceive things. I like to say that they make us more "real."

As Kyle's behavior changed, the conflict in our home eased. He felt better about himself and this was reflected in his daily interactions. As we became more "real" as a family, we found ourselves re-evaluating everything in our lives.

We felt we needed to re-examine how we chose to spend our time, our outside commitments and our hobbies and interests. This re-evaluation included our moving to a smaller home with a large yard for planting a garden and fruit trees. It also included a change in career for me, a shift in my husband's priorities and retirement plans and the decision to begin home schooling our boys. The raw food diet had allowed us to become more aligned with our essence. We were able to step back from the chaos of the world and experience an inner peace and harmony that we had not even been aware had been missing. We naturally gravitated toward what was natural and in this, we found ourselves very much "unplugging" from the world.

A major step in this "unplugging" was selling the T.V. in our living room. The constant barrage of fast–food commercials, superficial values and materialistic messages that came into our home became unacceptable. At first, we began to restrict the boys to a few hours per week but, even this amount of T.V. viewing proved insidious, causing a ripple in our otherwise peaceful household whenever they would watch it. When we finally decided to cut out the T.V. watching "cold turkey" (I must admit my husband Clyde was the last holdout for this decision), the change in our boys was wonderful. The first two days they had "withdrawal," complaining of boredom and acting pretty miserable. But, after two days time, they began to actually interact and *play* with each other. (I know you parents of siblings who are three years apart in age can appreciate what a revelation this was.)

Their imaginations kicked in, they built things, created art projects and wrote stories. The more they "unplugged" from the outside influences, the more "real" they became and the more peaceful our home became. We did keep a small T.V. in our back bedroom. This is used on rare occasions (the rental of a family movie or a favorite Star Trek episode) but, even those times are becoming less and less frequent as we now spend more time together as a family, playing games, reading stories or just talking. We didn't expect a change in diet to reach into every aspect of our lives, but once your body is allowed to return to a natural state of balance, your outside world must follow suit. The raw food diet is definitely a powerful transformational tool.

I felt it important to share these changes with you because the changes you implement in your child's diet have the potential to transform every aspect of your lives, especially if you are successful in transitioning your entire family to a raw food lifestyle. Take your time, these changes come at their own pace, in the natural order of things. Focus on putting pure, natural food in and nature will take it from there.

Chapter 7
Meal Ideas

When we first began our raw food journey I exhausted myself. I approached raw food meals as I always had cooked food meals. I tried to duplicate the dishes and variations we were used to in an attempt to get my family to eat this way. We tried two or three raw food dishes every night. This was an incredible amount of work. Since it was new to me, it made it seem even more difficult. I soon realized this wasn't the way it was supposed to be and I had to change my idea of what meals should be.

We, as parents, are used to preparing meals for our children with basic food groups in mind. There is usually a main dish (meat, or a protein source if you are a vegetarian), a starch and a vegetable. This is how we learned to cook. As a raw foodist you can forget all that. Simplicity is the key. It is perfectly alright (even optimal) to sit down and eat three bananas for lunch. If you make the preparation of raw food meals into work, you have missed the point. This is especially important if there are others in your household who are not following a raw food diet.

If you are trying to prepare two different meals for your family's dinner, you are setting yourself up for disaster. Try to get away from the idea that each meal has to be different.

Once the body is cleansed, salad tastes wonderful every day. It's only in the beginning that you crave other things. As the impurities are cleaned out of your body, they circulate in the bloodstream, producing cravings for these substances. Once pure, you will no longer have these cravings and will be satisfied with fresh fruits and vegetables. Keep this in mind as you transition your child. He will crave the old foods too. Realize what is happening and know that it does pass.

The following examples will give you some idea of what a raw family eats on any given day. There are also some ideas for each meal and some tips on how to incorporate raw items into your menus if you have other household members who are not eating as you are. By slowly increasing the raw items and decreasing the cooked items, your family will gradually transition to a predominately raw food diet.

Breakfast

The idea that breakfast is the most important meal of the day comes from the advertising of the cereal companies. It's actually better to have only juice or fruit until the noon meal, or to skip breakfast altogether, allowing the body to continue it's fast (detoxification) which began during the night. A heavy breakfast ties up the body's energy, making us sluggish and tired. In the morning, we usually have vegetable juice which I make in the Champion Juicer. This includes carrot, apple, kale, celery, and just about anything I have in the refrigerator. Sometimes we substitute fresh squeezed citrus, depending on the season. Clyde feels he needs something more substantial in the morning and usually has some manna bread or sprouted buckwheat as a cereal with his juice.

Kyle usually opts for sliced fruit or sprouted buckwheat cereal with raisins. Zack, my oldest son, prefers only juice for breakfast and has a mid-morning snack of fruit as he gets hungry. Alternatively, you could serve cut melon, a smoothie, fresh berries in the summer or soaked, dried fruit in winter.

Lunch

At lunch, I let my boys decide if they want fruit or a green salad. They choose what appeals to them at that time (translation—they choose what their body tells them they need). Kyle usually chooses a green salad. Zack chooses heavier foods like banana and apple, sometimes dipped in raw almond butter. Clyde prefers a fruit salad at lunch and I usually have one or two pieces of fruit, depending on what appeals to me at the time.

In Chapter 3, I discussed ideas for school lunches. If your family is eating lunch at home the choices are broader. If they are not yet totally raw you can provide a bowl of vegetable soup or some steamed vegetables. The most difficult thing is to wean them away from the typical lunchtime sandwich. Cooked starch (bread) is one of the most difficult addictions to give up. I refer to cooked starch as an addiction because I believe the chemical reaction within our bodies to eating cooked starch acts as a drug, provoking a sort of sedative effect. This has been my own experience after going for some time without bread, then eating it again. If you doubt the addictive quality of bread, try this experiment yourself. You can substitute manna bread (not a raw food) if you wish, or make a wrap from a cabbage or lettuce leaf (roll up your choice of vegetables; avocado, sprouts, cucumber, tomato, grated zucchini, etc.).

Dinner

This is where it gets tricky. Families typically go their own way throughout the day but, come together for dinner. For this reason, dinner seems more "official" and carries more meaning as we prepare the food we are to share with our loved ones. You can use this to your advantage as you enlist the help of your child. Have him help prepare the evening salad, taking care to arrange everything attractively and talking about the foods you are serving. This can be a special one–on–one time for you and your children.

Dinner in our house is usually a large salad. We may vary that two or three nights a week with raw zucchini "pasta" or a sea vegetable salad. The boys always have salad with us and two nights a week will also have a baked potato or yam. Once a week they will have a plate of lightly steamed vegetables or soup (split pea, broccoli, potato or vegetable) with their salad.

If there are members of your household who are not following the raw food diet you can always make a large salad to share with everyone and serve a cooked vegetarian entree (such as listed above). There are many different types of salads to choose from, even some familiar favorites (coleslaw, carrot raisin, marinated cucumbers, etc.). Be sure to always serve something raw along with the cooked foods.

Dessert

Like all kids, mine love dessert. I used to make raw desserts several times a week but found the involved recipes too time consuming. Now, we will have a raw pie or dehydrated cookies on special occasions only. The remainder of the time, if we want dessert (usually one to two hours after our evening meal), we simply eat a few dates or a banana with fruit sauce. Sometimes I make banana ice cream in the Champion Juicer (run frozen bananas through the juicer with the solid plate in place) or Kyle makes his specialty; banana, split lengthwise, spread with almond butter, topped with raisins.

Snacks

Snacks are anytime you are hungry! Some days my boys want to eat all day, like one long snack! A piece of fruit is a great snack, easy to carry, no packaging and provides quick energy. My boys also like dates (they think of them as candy), nuts (almonds are Kyle's favorite), dried fruit leather, celery sticks with raw nut butter, smoothies and homemade banana ice cream and sorbets. Before we were raw foodists, I was always wary of what the kids ate for snacks. I didn't want them to fill up on snacks before a meal, thinking they wouldn't have room for the healthier foods that were to come. Now, I don't mind what or when they eat. I know their snacks are just as healthy as their meals. When you are eating pure food, in it's natural state, there is no need to call it breakfast, lunch or dinner. It's simply nutrition the body needs and is appropriate anytime you're hungry.

Is it Expensive?

I am often asked about the cost of feeding a family a predominately raw diet. We all know the importance of eating organic, but the cost of organic produce can be prohibitive, especially when feeding a family. Availability is another concern. In certain areas of the country, organic produce is not readily available, especially in the winter months.

I practice the old adage "accept what you cannot change" when it comes to organic produce. The items that are relatively inexpensive and we eat a lot of (lettuce, tomatoes, juicing carrots, apples, cucumbers, celery, kale), I always buy organic. I am fortunate to live in Northern California, and am able to find these items year round. Other organic items I order by mail (dates, olives, sprouting seeds, beans and grains). I have included these distributors in the resources section. Items such as non-seasonal fruits, avocados, some nuts and dried fruit I buy non–organic. In the summer, having a garden definitely helps the grocery bill, providing organic, fresh, ready to eat produce just steps from your door. Over all, for our family of four, we spend anywhere from $500 to $600 per month on groceries, depending on the season. Since we home school, the children eat all their meals at home and Clyde takes his lunch to work. Because we juice, I buy our carrots and apples organic. I estimate this to be a cost of approximately $35 to $50 per month, depending on the cost of organic carrots. I did find that early on, when we were still buying half cooked food items and half raw items, we spent almost $900 per month. That was during the time I was heavily into preparing raw recipes and trying something new every day. The cost of fresh foods (even organic) is still considerably lower than processed and convenience foods. The cost of packaging (cans, bottles, boxes, freezer packs, etc.) is costly to the pocketbook and the planet. Buy in bulk when possible (sprouting grains and seeds, nuts and dried fruit, fresh fruit in season), buy organic when feasible and adjust your diet to accommodate the available fresh produce.

Chapter 8
Helpful Equipment

I want to make it clear that there is no special equipment necessary to succeed on a raw food diet. All we need to eat our natural diet and be healthy is what we came into this world with. Please do not feel you need to buy any or all of these appliances to be successful in transitioning your child. It's easy to go overboard with them and end up spending more time in the kitchen than you did before you were raw!

However, we are a society used to kitchen gadgets, convenience and a large variety of food textures and tastes. Because of this, having a few kitchen appliances can make the transition easier. The following are the appliances I use and what I mainly use them for.

Dehydrator – I have the Excalibur Dehydrator, 9 tray model. They are also available in 4 or 5 tray models. The Excalibur dehydrator has an adjustable thermostat (85° to 145°), which allows you to dehydrate well below the temperature where enzymes are destroyed. Prior to the Excalibur, I had an American Harvest Dehydrator. This model had no thermostat and didn't dry as efficiently or evenly as the Excalibur. I use the dehydrator to make dehydrated crackers, cookies or nut/seed burgers. In the summer when the garden is full, I use it to dry herbs for storage, and to dry summer harvest fruit for the winter.

<u>Champion Juicer</u> – We make juice almost every morning in our Champion. It juices hard vegetables well (carrot, apples, celery, beets, cumbers, broccoli, etc.). Greens are not it's forte, although it will do a few greens if pushed through with a carrot or apple. In addition, the Champion has a solid plate that enables you to make wonderful frozen desserts from frozen fruit. A few of our favorites are banana ice cream, frozen mango pie, watermelon sorbet, strawberry parfait and orange sherbet. Using the solid plate, the Champion will also grind nuts into nut butters and make a paste of soaked nuts and/or seeds to be used for pate or dehydrated crackers or burgers.

<u>Vita–Mix Blender</u> – The Vita–Mix is a very powerful blender. It will make juice from fresh fruits and vegetables, frozen ice creams from frozen fruit, blend vegetables into soup and make fresh smoothies from fresh and frozen fruit. We use it almost every day; smoothies, raw hummus, raw marinara sauce from sun dried tomatoes, raw pesto, raw cranberry sauce, frozen banana ice cream and blended soups. (Which the Vita–Mix will actually heat slightly as it blends, providing a warmed soup without heating enough to kill the enzymes.) I have had mine about 5 years and it's still going strong.

<u>Food Processor</u> – I use a Cuisinart Food Processor. Of the appliances I've listed, I use this the least. I have found it useful for making raw dips, crusts for raw pie by

processing nuts and dates together and processing seeds for dehydrated crackers. It's more effective than the Vita–Mix when processing items that are lacking in moisture (nuts, seeds, etc.). Wet items do not process as well as the liquid tends to run up and out the sides.

Saladacco Spiralizer – This is a handy, inexpensive gadget that allows you to make raw "pasta" from hard vegetables, such as zucchini. It's very easy to use and to clean. You simply place the vegetable in the holder and manually turn the crank. For transition, try substituting raw zucchini "pasta" for spaghetti noodles and top with your child's favorite marinara sauce. Traditional pasta is void of taste until you put the sauce on it anyway, they may not even notice!

Water Filter – We have a reverse–osmosis water filter in our kitchen, which was professionally installed and fits under our sink. I highly recommend you use some type of water filter and/or distiller for your drinking (and sprout and nut soaking) water. The additives and impurities in our country's drinking water makes this of utmost importance.

Chapter 9
Cautions and Concerns

I felt it was necessary for this revised edition to include this chapter. There is little information available for parents who wish to raise their children on the raw food diet and as a result much is learned through trial and error. Unfortunately, there are few success stories and most that I have heard of are regarding older children, not babies raised from birth on a raw food diet.

Over the past four years, since the first release of *Raw Kids*, I have counseled many parents who were having problems of one sort or another as they attempted to transition their children. The vast majority of these problems were concerning toddlers and younger children. The thing they all had in common was being too strict and ridged with the diet. One mother I spoke with had created a power play between her five year old son and herself which was acted out every night at dinner. He wanted some cooked foods and she refused to allow him to have any at all. Soon he rejected everything she offered him and he became angry and aggressive toward her. The stress this was causing her family far outweighed any physical detriment the cooked food might have caused. She had lost perspective about what is important, focusing only on the food, as if her son was a one-dimensional being, rather than a multi-faceted unique individual.

Another mother confided that her two-year old son (who had been raw since birth), was showing signs of abnormal development and deficiencies. His teeth were a greenish-yellow color as they came in (lack of calcium), he was listless and "blank" much of the time and he was underweight and below average in height. He had these symptoms even though he was still being breastfed. This mother was very knowledgeable in the area of raw foods, having been 100% raw herself for many years. She knew all the right things to feed her son and was very careful with his diet. His failure to thrive finally convinced her to include some cooked foods in his diet. When she did this, he immediately began to improve in every area. Soon, he was an alert and active toddler and he quickly gained weight. This experience made her reconsider her own dietary habits and change her ridged view of the "optimal" diet.

Besides being too ridged, the next mistake many parents make is not listening to their own inner knowing with regard to their children's diets. They unquestionably follow what the "experts" say, not realizing that most teachers in the raw food movement do not have children so, their advice exists only in theory, not actual practice with tangible results. One such case is a mother who contacted me frantic because her four year old daughter was so weak she could hardly stand. She had been fasting the child, under the advice of a natural-health physician (not an M.D.) to rid the child of a skin rash. The guidance had been via telephone, he had never physically examined the child. He specialized in raw food diets and used fasting as a "cure" for just about everything. The fast had lasted nearly a week with no improvement in the rash. When she became worried that her daughter was getting too weak she phoned him again, asking him what to do. He advised her to continue the fast for another three to five days! Even though this went against all her material instincts, she was going along with his advice. It was then that she remembered reading my book and contacted me for advice and support. I urged her to listen to her heart and to give her daughter some juice and then gradually introduce solid food again. (For further information, see the section below on detoxification).

Children lose nutrients very quickly as they have little or no reserves. Except in very rare instances, a child this young should not be fasted. If they are fasted at all it should only be under the direct, physical supervision of a professional physician. At the very least, this woman should have consulted an M.D. but, she was so trusting of this man's advice, believing he was an "expert", she ignored her instincts which told her to stop the fast and give her daughter some food.

No one knows your child like you do. You must trust your instincts. Even if something has worked for others, that does not mean it is right for your child. Educate yourself as best you can, then apply that knowledge to your own situation. Children are growing and changing in so many different ways (physical, emotional, etc.). What worked yesterday may not work today. Be creative and don't be afraid to fail, the only failure is to not learn from one's experiences.

Children have different needs than adults. The knowledge you have through your own experience with the raw food diet may not follow for your children. Below are some specific areas which are different for children than adults.

Detoxification

Because their bodies are usually more efficient, children detoxify at a very rapid rate. I do not believe a child under ten should be purposefully fasted for any reason (this refers to a complete fast where only water is given, a diet of juice only for a few days may be acceptable under certain conditions). The reason is that children have a much cleaner system than adults, lacking the years of dietary indiscretions and environmental pollution that most adults have been subjected to. Children also have less nutrient stores than adults and therefore become depleted more rapidly. A child who goes without food for several days will become depleted much more rapidly than an adult.

Children are much more tuned into the natural rhythm of their bodies because they lack the indoctrination most adults have had with regard to diet and health. They follow their natural tendencies much more readily than adults. In nature, one can observe animals fasting through instinct alone. They instinctively know when they are not well and their bodies tell them not to eat. Children have the same ability if we will only listen. If they don't want to eat, they should not be made to. Allow them to follow their body's natural tendencies and teach them to trust in the natural rhythm of their body. If they can do that, detoxification will take care of itself.

Calories

Children need more calories than adults. There are great physiological demands on the body of a growing child. One must be careful when implementing changes which reduce or restrict caloric intake for children. Getting enough calories on a raw food diet is difficult for children, especially over the long term. During the time our family was totally raw, our boys lost a lot of weight, it got to the point where our relatives became concerned. At that point, they were nine and twelve years old and I was including a lot of high fat foods in their diet (avocados, nut and seed butters, young coconut meat and coconut milk) and they ate virtually non-stop because they were always hungry. As they grew and entered puberty, it became obvious that they were not thriving on a 100% raw diet and I began to lighten up on the strict idealism which pervades the raw food movement. This change coincided with my own raw food journey, explained in the next chapter, Intuitive Eating.

Behavioral Issues

It is well known that food is a source of comfort. It is grounding and makes us feel comfortable in our surroundings. Food acts as the energetic "bridge" through which the soul maintains the physical body that interacts with the physical world. When heavier foods are consumed, there is a dampening in the energetic field, which tends to keep energy from moving through the person's subtle bodies. When lighter foods are consumed, there is a lightening in the energetic field, which allows energies which have been stuck (we call this karma) to be released. That's one of the main reasons it is so difficult to stick to a lighter diet. It requires us to learn to process our suppressed emotions, insecurities, pain and fear.

When making a change to a lighter diet, whether it be vegetarianism, veganism or raw foodism, one may experience this release of energies in the form of heightened emotions, insecure feelings, aggressive tendencies, depression or anxiety which may alternate with feelings of elation and expansion. Each extreme will be intensified. With children, this can be especially frightening as they lack the maturity to process energies which have been carried forward from their soul's previous experiences.

This is another reason it is better to transition in a gradual way, rather than try and change everything at once. Be patient and give your child time to adjust energetically to what is happening physically. Erratic emotions and increased insecurity are signs that the transition should be slowed to allow the child to stabilize in small increments.

Keeping it in Perspective

Raising happy, healthy kids is much more than diet. Wellness needs to be addressed on many different levels. Helping your children learn to make their own choices, and allowing them to learn from those choices is the hardest thing for a parent to do but, it is necessary. Examine your motives for this dietary change, always veer toward the conservative side as this will minimize any physical and emotional difficulties which may arise. Never take your child's reaction as a failure on your part. Each soul has free will, a mind of his own and his own individual karmic pattern which is to be fulfilled for his life. Understand that teaching him about the choices that are available and helping him to learn about the consequences of those choices (such as dietary indiscretions) is more important than controlling every aspect of his diet. This is unconditional love, the most important thing you can give your child. Rather than viewing foods as "right or wrong", "good or bad", help your child understand there are simply different choices available to him and let him discover what each choice feels like on his own. Someday he will be on his own, having to make his own choices in a world full of indiscretions. If he has confidence in himself and confidence in his own decisions, he will surely carry all you have taught him throughout his life.

Summary

I have included this chapter and the examples of problems encountered with the raw food diet, not to dissuade you, but to bring into the open that which is seldom spoken of in the raw food movement. So often these problems are glossed over or omitted entirely, as if they do not or should not happen. My experience and that of countless parents whom I have been in contact with, prove these problems do exist and are very common.

Many raw food teachers would have you believe that everyone is better off on a 100% raw food diet and if any difficulties are encountered, you are simply doing something wrong. As for children, there is little to no direct experience to draw upon in the raw food movement as a whole and parents are left to their own devices, trying to do what is best for their children and fighting the fear that they may be inadvertently doing some harm.

There is no question that nearly everyone can benefit from a lighter diet. Bringing awareness into this area is a huge step in the right direction. I do feel that moderation is best with regard to children and that the focus should be on teaching them about food and the choices available, rather than being ridged and worrying about every morsel they put in their mouths. Eventually, you will need to find a balance that works for your child and your family's lifestyle. No one can tell you what that is. You may settle on a vegetarian diet, a vegan diet, a predominately raw food diet or even a total raw food diet, perhaps fluctuating at different times throughout the year. In actuality, we are always in a state of transition because we are multidimensional beings and our physical needs fluctuate according to many factors (environment, emotional, hormonal, age, gender, attitude, belief structure, and even energetic fluctuations which occur on the non-physical level and affect us all planetarily to varying degrees). Therefore, dietary transition should be viewed as an on-going process rather than a means to an end.

I believe that initially, most people are attracted to the raw food diet as a means of bringing more simplicity and peace into their lives. They are seeking harmony with the earth and with creation. They are rebelling against the materialistic and superficial attitudes and structures of a society which has lost it's balance and it's connection to creation. It is rarely about the diet itself, but about an overall change in focus and lifestyle. Understanding this will help you find balance and give you perspective through the changes a dietary transition brings. Raising a well-adjusted, confident child who is not afraid to explore, ask for forgiveness and learn from his mistakes, requires that you also need to be confident, be willing to explore, ask for forgiveness and learn from your mistakes. It is a journey that spans many lifetimes...

Update

Currently, (four years after our initial raw food transition) my boys are eating a diet consisting of 50% raw and living foods and 50% cooked foods consisting of vegetables, grains and some fish. We also regularly include soy meat substitutes, tofu and raw milk.

We have come to a peaceful balance and the boys have learned so much through this process. Neither one will touch meat and are known throughout their school as the "resident vegetarians" (the only ones in their school). They read labels, observe their peers eating habits and understand why wise food choices are important. They are thriving and have grown into well-adjusted, happy young men.

Although, we did not stick with 100% raw foods, I am happy with how our journey has evolved. We have achieved a wonderful and peaceful balance, one which allows for a healthy lifestyle, while still allowing freedom to participate socially in the world. (See chapter 10, *Intuitive Eating* for more details on our raw food journey.) If one is too different, there is a separation which occurs with one's peers, whether they be children or adults. This became very evident as the boys reached their teenage years. The raw food diet and lifestyle should be taught to children as an option, one that they can choose on their own if they so desire. Every seed planted will remain, holding the potential to sprout at the optimum time.

Chapter 10
Intuitive Eating

This chapter first appeared as an article in Get Fresh! magazine in May, 2003. I have included it due to the many inquiries I have received over the years. You will not be able to help your child change his eating habits until you come to terms with your own issues in this area. You must feel peaceful within yourself or your child will sense your ambiguity. Every transition is a learning experience for everyone involved however, it is necessary to set an example for your child or they will not respond favorably to any change you try and implement. It is my sincere wish that my shared experience below will assist you as you seek to find resolution and balance within yourself and your family.

I was first led to raw foods in the early stages of my Kundalini process and I found it to be an excellent way to purify and detoxify the body and spirit. When the body is lighter (vibrationally) and as the consciousness becomes lighter, you are better able to perceive and experience the Kundalini energy. Like so many others, I thought I had discovered the long-lost secret of all secrets and I was absolutely positive that following a 100% raw food diet was the remedy for the ails of mankind.

As my Kundalini process progressed, I began to delve more deeply into the spiritual teachings of the enlightened Sages, Masters and Gurus. I used to wonder why, these enlightened beings, who had the wisdom and benefit of higher states of consciousness and expanded human awareness, did not mention the raw food diet in their teachings? How could they not know about the raw food diet? How could they not see this truth that appeared so obvious to me? Why did they not follow the raw food diet themselves? How could they reach such a perfected state of consciousness without the benefit of the one and only true diet for mankind? These questions plagued me and as I entered the latter stages of the Kundalini process and began to access these higher states of consciousness for myself, I began to understand.

What these Masters knew was that while it was certainly preferable to eat a vegetarian diet which includes plenty of fresh fruits and vegetables, balance is the most important ingredient for any level of higher awareness to be realized and stabilized through the human vehicle. Balance being essential to the Kundalini process, I soon discovered that to achieve balance required flexibility. As the Kundalini ascended into the higher chakras and my energetic body became more integrated into my physical body, I was unable to continue with a predominately raw diet. I was not able to stabilize the energy until I added back in some cooked food such as steamed vegetables, tofu, steamed rice, vegetarian soups, etc. I experimented a lot and listened to my body on a daily basis. What prompted this change was that I began having a lot of trouble with my intestines (bloating, indigestion, constipation), which I didn't understand. As I asked about this, I intuitively received an answer to read a book about the Ayurveda system, an ancient Vedic system of health care which classifies body types (called doshas). I took the test in the book and found out I am predominately a vata type, which is the most sensitive constitutional type and also the easiest to upset and throw into imbalance.

When I read about vata imbalance, I knew that was what had happened to me. The symptoms and my experience fit exactly. I was shocked to learn that the recommended diet for vata is minimal raw foods! The basic constitutional elements of a vata type are air and ether. Therefore, the increased energy (prana) that was flooding my system, added to my already energetically charged and light constitution, really threw me into chaos, having no elements to ground or balance my physical body. I immediately started implementing the suggestions in the book and my intestinal problems were gone in three days!

Having been heavily into the raw food movement, I was well aware of the school of thought that one can balance a vata constitution on a raw food diet by exercising more care with regard to the preparation and types of raw foods. I attempted this several times without much success. From that point on, I learned to listen to my body on a daily basis. I no longer relied on any specific preset dietary guidelines, including the Ayurveda system. I realized that the Kundalini process was being directed by a higher intelligence and that the existing dietary guidelines and various dietary regimens had not been created for someone experiencing the extreme physiological and energetic transformation of the Kundalini process. I understood my body had a whole new set of needs, and I began to trust the Divine, through the wisdom of my body itself, for my nutritional guidance.

My experience has required that I change my belief that the raw food diet is always the right diet for everyone, all of the time. I have had many clients who have come to me with physical and emotional problems resulting from the raw food diet. While they often times experienced wonderful and dramatic results at first, as time went on, they found it increasingly difficult to live up to the ridged and idealistic standards presented by most of the raw food teachers. Feeling disheartened, they reverted back to their old eating habits, usually after many months of inner conflict and feelings of failure.

On several occasions, in my capacity as a Medical Intuitive, I have been consulted by people who had developed severe physical problems as a result of the rigidity of the raw food diet. One such woman, who also has active Kundalini, had been advised by a raw food educator to omit every source of fat from her diet. This suggestion was made in an attempt to clear up her Candida problem. Because she was trying to follow a vegan, raw-foot diet, omitting all the fat also meant omitting the major sources of protein (nuts, seeds and their butters). The result was that within one month, she developed severe symptoms of MS (Muscular Dystrophy). These symptoms sent her to her allopathic doctor for a battery of tests, all of which came out negative. As I intuitively scanned her body, it appeared that the nerve sheaths were "raw" resulting from there being no conduct-ability through the nerve pathways of her nervous system. Nerve impulses were being sent by her brain, but were not flowing to the nerve endings. The resultant symptoms were tingling and numbness in her limbs. The increased activity of the Kundalini energy through her nervous system required her to eat more fat and protein to allow the nervous system to keep up with the added demands of the intense physiological changes of the Kundalini process. Her nervous system was starving for fat! When she did not give her body what it wanted, physical damage was the result. She said she had been craving flax seed oil (fat) and eggs (protein) so badly she could barely stand it but was fighting these cravings because she was trying to stick to the raw food diet as strictly prescribed. Her body was suffering, her psyche was suffering, her self-esteem and inner-peace were suffering while her medical bills were increasing! How simple it would have been for her to just "give into" what her body was craving! I realize this is an extreme example. Most people do not have active Kundalini nor the extreme physiological demands this process brings. This is an excellent example however, of the varying needs which arise within our bodies on a constant basis and the need to honor what our bodies are telling us. The strict idealism of the raw food movement is not conducive to achieving a healthy balance through increased awareness of the process of intuitive eating. When one begins on the raw food path, it is very common to be told that all difficulties that arise are due to detoxification and that they will subside over time. So much of the movement focuses only on the physical aspects. People are taught what to eat, how to prepare (or not to prepare) the food, what to expect through detoxification, etc. They read and re-read the raw food success stories and look to the raw food teachers as role models. When one encounters difficulty and it becomes difficult to strictly follow the raw food path, what was once a joyous expression of life becomes a source of conflict.

Success on the raw food path or in any endeavor depends on balance. To achieve balance requires awareness of all the variables. Through that awareness, we evolve into greater self-mastery. When we focus only on the physical aspects of the raw food diet, we are leaving out several very important variables. In addition to the physical body, we have an emotional body, a spiritual body, an astral body and a mental body. You are a multi-dimensional being and every aspect of your being directly affects and interacts with every other aspect. There are a myriad of energies at work in and through the individual and planetary consciousness at all times. You cannot escape these influences. Even if you are not interested in anything beyond the physical practicalities of your diet, you are still being affected by these variables. To ignore them creates imbalance.

Once my Kundalini process completed, I found my body once again changing what it wanted in order to bring balance. I was again drawn to lighter foods and began eating mostly raw, fresh foods. I still eat occasional fish, range-free eggs, raw milk, tofu and sprouted, whole grain bread because my body craves them and is thriving. I am aware of the more subtle levels of my being and can sense the interaction between the physical body and these other levels. I have learned to listen to what my body wants on any given day and I watch in awe and amazement at the wisdom it demonstrates as it works to establish balance at each level. As I encounter and stabilize higher and more refined states of consciousness, it has become clear that the farther we evolve as a species, the more we must humble ourselves to be able to discover what we have yet to experience. To believe anything is the "ultimate truth" that applies to everyone at all times, is the height of spiritual arrogance.

You must learn to eat intuitively and to rely on your own body to tell you what it needs. There simply is no other way to bring balance. No one can tell you what the ideal diet is for you. There simply are too many variables and these variables change on a daily basis. To eat intuitively is to be in balance with all of creation. This is a given, because your body naturally seeks balance and it will tell you what it needs on any given day. To rely on your body's innate wisdom means that you must free yourself from dietary idealism. You cannot hold yourself to some set of strict guidelines if your body is telling you something different. To do so goes against the balance which is naturally trying to become established through all aspects of your being.

If you are thriving on the raw food diet, that is wonderful. If you are having difficulty, it does not mean you are doing anything wrong. You are not weak because you have cravings or because you feel you need to include some cooked foods in your diet. Establishing balance takes time and very few people are able to embark on the raw food diet and stick to it with no problems. Truthfully, there are very few long term success stories because the goal (to be 100% raw) has been set too high and the standards too ridged with little understanding beyond the physical level.Change only comes through love and acceptance. Each and every difficulty happens to assist us in gaining self-awareness and each and every difficulty ceases when we release the need to live up to external standards. Be patient with yourself, know that you are changing on many (unseen) levels and that these changes will affect the needs and responses of your physical body. Learn to live (and eat) intuitively because there is a higher intelligence guiding your existence, one which will guide you into peace, happiness, health and balance....if only you will trust it above all else.

(For more information on the Kundalini process, see Solomae's book, *Kundalini and the Evolution of Consciousness* Living Spirit Press, 2003).

Chapter 9
Recipes

As I said before, when we began our raw food journey I went overboard in the food preparation area. I bought many raw food recipe books and tried a different dish every night. This was exhausting and expensive! Another issue to consider is your family's expectations. If you introduce the raw food diet with a variety of raw concoctions, attempting to copy their favorite dishes in raw form for each meal, what will happen when you are no longer able to keep up this pace? Will they revert back to their cooked food habits? Will you decide it's just too much work?

A more sensible approach (and I speak from experience) is to try a few special raw dishes, perhaps once or twice a week. The rest of the time provide wonderful salads and ripe fruits to be eaten in their natural state. Focus on getting your family used to the simplicity and peace of the raw food diet. Teach them the ease of grabbing a banana or cutting a watermelon. Change your mind–set regarding what constitutes a meal and focus on simplicity. Teach your child to appreciate the subtle qualities of a fresh peach, smell the nectar, touch the outer fuzz, taste the juice and relish the texture as it melts it's way down the throat.

A word about recipes. It's wonderful to look through recipe books in the beginning to get ideas and get a feel for what is possible with raw foods. However, you will find it much easier if you begin to develop your own recipes, based on a few family favorites. Keep it simple! Too many ingredients are too time consuming and too expensive for everyday use. For those of us with families who expect a meal on the table every evening, it has to be simple or it just won't work in the long run. Experiment and find a few "staples" that your family likes, then make your own variations. The raw food lifestyle is about freedom, not complication.

The recipes that follow are my own creation, unless otherwise noted. I would like to thank Rose Lee Calabro for her permission to include recipes from her book, *Living in the Raw, Recipes for a Healthy Lifestyle.*

Please note: Many of these recipes call for the addition of Bragg Liquid Aminos as a salt substitute. This inclusion is entirely optional. If you feel the need to include salt, you may also use sea salt, soy sauce or Nama Shoyu, an organic, unpasteurized soy sauce by Gold Mine Natural Foods. I have found this product to be superior to Bragg Liquid Aminos in that I feel no adverse reaction (headache or dizziness) to it, as I do with the Bragg product. It is recommended that you gradually reduce the intake of these salt substitutes as you wean your family off the tastes of processed foods.

The Art of Salad

For a raw foodist, salad is an art form. Prior to becoming a raw foodist, I thought a salad consisted of iceberg lettuce and sliced tomato. How times have changed! Now, when we prepare wonderfully imaginative salads almost every night of the week, I enlist the help of my boys. When they create their own salads, they look at it in a whole different way. Kyle loves to decoratively place the vegetables around the plate and sprinkle the sprouts as he chooses. When he helps prepare the evening salad he even places items on his salad that he had previously refused to eat, and proceeds to eat them! Including your child in the food preparation will make it more likely he will eat what is prepared. It gives him choices and a feeling of importance; it empowers him. Give him this gift.

We make our salads on a large dinner plate so everything is spread out and there is room for many different things. First, we make a bed on the plate of greens. This is usually a variety of red leaf lettuce or romaine lettuce, spinach, Chinese cabbage (sometimes called napa cabbage), or kale. I usually include three of these. We then add "everything but the kitchen sink." The following items are usually included, but vary according to availability:

Sliced tomato or several cherry tomatoes
Sliced cucumber
Celery (sliced)
Carrot (grated and placed as a scoop on top of the greens)
Sugar snap peas (wonderful to eat right out of the bag)
Red Cabbage (coarsely chopped or grated)
Mung bean, lentil and alfalfa sprouts
Jicama (diced)
Zucchini (grated or sliced)
Broccoli or cauliflower florerts
Bok choy (chopped)
Mushrooms
Avocado (sliced)
Olives (sun ripened)
Sunflower or pumpkin seeds

With a salad like that it's hard to get bored! We vary the dressing we use, each of us has our favorites. I make many dressings from raw ingredients and buy organic bottled dressings made with cold-pressed oils. My children are fond of the line of dressings made by "Annie's Naturals" and "New Organics Co." When we eat out, we always take a bottle of dressing with us. An easy (and raw) dressing that most people like is Lemon Tahini Dressing made by mixing the following: ½ cup raw sesame tahini, ½ cup cold–pressed olive oil, ½ cup lemon juice and ½ to ¾ cup water. Blend all ingredients together and add water as needed.

Taco Salad

Make these on large individual dinner plates.

Chopped romaine lettuce (or any type of loose leaf lettuce)
Chopped tomato
Olives
Sliced cucumber
Sprouts of your choice

Place a large scoop of freshly made guacamole (recipe below) in the center and spoon fresh salsa of your choice over entire salad.

Easy Guacamole

2   avocados
2   T lemon juice (or more, to taste)
½   t sea salt or Nama Shoyu to taste
1   tomato, chopped (optional)
1   t chili powder

Mash avocados in a small bowl. Stir in remaining ingredients. Taste and adjust seasonings.

Sprouting

Sprouting is a great way to familiarize your child with growing his own food. It's fast, easy and inexpensive. They can literally watch the sprouts grow daily, then pick them just before dinner and add to their salad.

Sprouts are a living food. Prior to soaking, the seed has within it all the life–producing energy of the universe. A mighty oak tree springs forth from one small seed. When you soak (germinate) the seed, this life–giving energy is awakened out of dormancy and new life springs forth in the form of a small shoot we refer to as a sprout. The new sprouts are full of vitamins, minerals and enzymes. They are literally a nutritional powerhouse.

When I first attempted to grow sprouts it was very foreign to me. All the soaking and rinsing seemed complicated. The sprouting charts specified different instructions for each item to be sprouted and I felt overwhelmed. Don't be fooled, mother nature is not that fragile! If you can soak it and run some water over it, you can sprout it. Don't get hung up on following the sprouting charts exactly. In sprouting, you're simply providing the conditions for the seed, grain or bean to reproduce. If you throw a handful of seeds on the ground, come next spring, you will have new plants. Don't make it harder than it is. The soaking times are *approximate*, nothing happens if you are over or under the specified time. It won't be long until sprouting is second nature to you. You will be growing enzyme and nutrient rich sprouts, inexpensively supplementing your family's food supply and in the process, teaching self sufficiency to your children.

Just about any seed, nut or grain can be sprouted. The two main methods to sprout are the water method and the soil method. Most seeds and nuts are sprouted using the water method. Baby greens are grown by sprouting grains such as wheat and barley and seeds such as sunflower using the soil method. (For detailed instructions and specific soaking and sprouting times, please refer to the books listed in the Resources Section.)

There are several different ways to produce sprouts using the water method. Depending on what you're sprouting, you may prefer the bag method, jar method or basket method. I prefer the jar method. Sun Organic Farm (see Resource Section) carries an inexpensive sprouting jar and lid set that comes with screw on lids in three different mesh sizes for different size sprouts. You just rinse and set upside down to let the water drain. Alternatively, you can use wide–mouthed canning jars with cheesecloth over the opening, secured by a rubber band.

We have five sprouting jars that we rotate. We grow alfalfa sprouts, sunflower sprouts, bean sprouts (I use an organic bean mix of green, french and red lentils, whole peas, mung beans and aduki beans from Sun Organic Farms) and buckwheat sprouts for breakfast cereal.

Buckwheat Breakfast Cereal

Buckwheat is one of the softest grains. It's delightfully moist and sprouts quickly and easily. I sprout mine in a sprouting jar.

Begin by soaking ¾ cup raw hulled buckwheat groats (available at most natural food stores or by mail order from Sun Organic Farm) for 5 – 6 hours. Drain and rinse several times, until the water runs clear. Turn jar upside down in a dish drainer. Repeat this rinsing several times throughout the day. You will notice sprouts appearing after one day. Continue to rinse several times a day for two days (the sprouts will be about ¼ inch in length), they are now ready to eat. Place desired amount of sprouts in a bowl (it doesn't take much, they are dense and filling) and top with raisins or fruit of your choice. Add raw nut milk (almond, cashew, etc.) or commercial rice or soy milk. Alternatively, you could soak dried fruit overnight and when you add the fruit to the cereal, use the soak water to sweeten and moisten.

This is a good recipe for transition because it's filling and substitutes for the processed breakfast cereals so many children are used to. I store the sprouts (jar and all) in the refrigerator up to 3 days. The sprouts will continue to grow, but they may still be eaten.

Vegetable Crackers

We use these crackers as snacks, sometimes topped with raw nut butter, raw hummus, guacamole or salsa. This is a versatile recipe and I have made several variations, such as omitting some of the vegetables or using almonds or other seeds in place of the pumpkin seeds.

Recipe from *Living in the Raw*, by Rose Lee Calabro. Reprinted with permission.

1   cup sunflower seeds, soaked 6 – 8 hours and rinsed
1   cup pumpkin seeds, soaked 6 – 8 hours
2   carrots
1   red bell pepper, finely chopped
1   red onion, finely chopped
2   stalks celery, finely chopped
2   cloves garlic (optional)
¼   cup fresh parsley, finely chopped
1   T Bragg Liquid Aminos

Process sunflower seeds, pumpkin seeds and carrots through a Champion Juicer using the solid plate. Add red bell peppers, red onion, celery, garlic, parsley and Bragg. Form round crackers about 1 ½ in diameter and ¼ thick. Place on a dehydrator tray with teflex sheet. Dehydrate at 105° for 4 hours, flip crackers over, and remove teflex sheet. Continue dehydrating for 3–6 hours, or until desired crispness is obtained.

Raw Hummus

Raw hummus is a wonderful dip for raw vegetables or spread for dehydrated crackers or Essene bread. You can add as much tahini as you like, creating a smoother texture. Be sure to process thoroughly to obtain the creamiest texture.

2 cups sprouted chickpeas* (also called garbanzo beans)
¼ cup fresh–squeezed lemon juice
1 T minced garlic (optional)
½ cup raw tahini
¼ cup olive oil
Nama Shoyu (or other salt substitute) to taste

Blend all ingredients in a food processor or blender until creamy.

* To sprout chickpeas: Soak chickpeas 24 – 48 hours (the longer the soak time the easier the digestion). Drain water and let sprout for 2 days, rinsing three times a day. (¾ cup dry chickpeas will yield approximately 2 cups sprouted).

Marinated Vegetable Salad

An easy make–ahead salad, good for those busy days. Use any vegetables you have on hand. A nice addition is to sprinkle clover or alfalfa sprouts on the salad before serving.

1   bunch broccoli, chopped into florets
1   cup fresh corn kernels
4   scallions, finely minced
1   garlic clove (optional)
4   T olive oil
¼   cup lemon juice
     sea salt or Nama Shoyu to taste

Mix all ingredients in a large bowl. Refrigerate for at least 20 minutes, toss and serve.

Spinach Sprout Salad

This is one of my favorites. It gets a wonderful "zing" from the sun–dried tomatoes and is a good way to incorporate more sprouts and dark leafy greens into a child's diet. For added zing, add some sliced green olives.

Combine the following in a large bowl:

1   head red leaf or romaine lettuce torn into bite size pieces
1   bunch spinach – coarsely chopped
1   zucchini – sliced ¼" thick, then quartered
1   cup small sprouts (alfalfa or clover work well)
½   cup sun–dried tomatoes (soak in water for 3 hours then drain and chop)
¼   cup chopped fresh basil or ½ tsp dried

Dressing

Combine the following in a small bowl, mix well with a fork and pour over salad.

¼   cup cold–pressed olive oil
3   T lemon juice
½   t Dijon style mustard (omit for 100% raw dressing)
1   clove minced garlic
1   T Nama Shoyu or sea salt to taste

Kale Salad

A fast, easy salad. It's especially good when you have time to make it ahead and let it sit for an hour or more.

Combine the following in a large bowl:

1   bunch kale (stem removed), rinsed and chopped
2   tomatoes, chopped (or one cup cherry tomatoes)
¼   cup pumpkin seeds

Dressing:

3   T olive oil
3   T lemon juice
1   T water
1   clove garlic (minced)
1   T Nama Shoyu

Combine dressing ingredients in a measuring cup and mix until frothy. Pour over salad, mix and serve.

Raw Pasta Sauce

Use this sauce over raw zucchini "pasta" made with the Saladacco (see page 51).

1   cup sun dried tomatoes - If using bagged dried to-
    matoes, soak in water for 2 hours and keep the soak
    water. If using tomatoes packed in oil, reduce or
    eliminate the olive oil from the recipe. Chop them
    coarsely and put in blender.
1   cup fresh chopped tomatoes
½   cup fresh basil leaves
2   tsp soy sauce, Nama Shoyu or sea salt to taste
3   garlic cloves - minced
¼   cup pine nuts (optional)
¼   cup cold-pressed olive oil (omit if using dried toma-
    toes packed in oil)
¼   cup water (if using tomatoes soaked in water, use
    the soak water) add a little at a time, more or
    less for desired consistency.

Place all ingredients in a blender and blend on the low
setting or pulse. Don't puree, you want some chunks
left in it, like pasta sauce. Better to under-process than
over-process. Add water as needed. Spoon over "pasta"
and serve. If desired, you can warm this sauce over a
very low heat, being careful not to heat past the tepid
stage (it should be slightly warm to your finger) before
serving.

Apple Carrot Salad

A festive, colorful salad. We like to serve this on holidays or special occasions.

Recipe from *Living in the Raw*, by Rose Lee Calabro. Reprinted with permission.

1   apple, cored and grated
2   carrots, grated
½   cup currants
½   cup orange juice
2   T lemon juice
1   T lemon zest
1   ½ t grated fresh ginger
¼   cup walnuts, soaked 6 – 8 hours, chopped
1   T shredded coconut

Combine apple, carrots, currants, orange juice, lemon zest, and ginger. Stir in walnuts and coconut just before serving.

Smoothies

Smoothies are a staple in our house. Every smoothie is different. Using whatever fresh fruit you have on hand, you can create these luscious treats anytime. Try one for breakfast!

Basic Smoothie Recipe

Blend the following ingredients and serve:

1   cup fresh fruit (berries, banana, pear, mango, strawberries, pineapple, etc.)
½   cup frozen fruit (strawberries, mango, banana, etc.) add 3 – 6 dates if you like it sweeter water or fruit juice to reach desired consistency.

Variations:

Substitute ¼ cup cashews or almonds and ½ cup water (this creates nut milk) for the water or fruit juice.

Add a tablespoon of tahini. (Tahini is high in calcium and adds beneficial fat and calories for active children).

"Chocolate" Shake

This smoothie tastes like a chocolate milkshake. Guaranteed to satisfy a sweet tooth or chocolate craving!

Blend the following ingredients and serve:

1   fresh banana
1   frozen banana
4   pitted dates (more or less, depending on how sweet you want it)
1   T raw carob powder (available at natural food stores)
1   cup water (more or less depending on the consistency you want)
1   T raw tahini (optional)

Banana Coconut Salad

This is a good lunchtime salad. Make it in the morning and pack in a container for school lunches. The orange juice will keep the bananas fresh for 4 – 5 hours.

6 bananas – sliced
1 pint blueberries
¼ cup flaked unsweetened coconut
½ cup chopped walnuts (soaked 8 hours)
½ cup fresh squeezed orange juice

Combine sliced bananas, coconut and chopped walnuts in a bowl. Stir in orange juice and serve.

Variation: Substitute sliced strawberries or chopped pineapple for the blueberries.

Fruit Sauces

These fruit sauces are wonderful to pour over sliced or chopped fruit. They provide a change of pace that makes fruit salad seem like an elegant treat. They are fast and easy to make and keep for several days in the refrigerator.

Banana Strawberry Sauce

Blend the following ingredients and serve:

1 fresh banana
4 large strawberries
2 dates (optional, for added sweetness)

Pour over sliced fruit and top with chopped walnuts.

Cranberry Sauce

This is one of our favorites. Try it over sliced bananas for a taste treat.

Recipe by Rose Lee Calabro. Reprinted with Permission.

2 cups fresh cranberries
1 orange
1 apple
1 cup dates
water for desired consistency

Process cranberries, orange, apple and dates in a blender until smooth. Pour over fruit or eat as is.

"Chocolate" Sauce

Blend the following ingredients and serve:

½ cup raw cashews
1 cup water
4 pitted dates (more or less, depending on desired sweetness)
1 fresh banana
2 T raw carob powder

Pour over sliced banana and sprinkle with flaked unsweetened coconut. This is a very elegant dessert.

Apple Raisin Cookies

Recipe from *Living in the Raw*, by Rose Lee Calabro. Reprinted with permission. Rose Lee says this is one of her favorites. (My kids like them too!) This recipe was also featured in Veggie Life Magazine.

2 cups sunflower seeds, soaked 6 – 8 hours and rinsed
2 Fuji apples
2 large bananas
½ cup honey dates
1 t vanilla
1 t cinnamon
1 cup raisins
1 cup walnuts, soaked 6 – 8 hours and chopped

Process sunflower seeds, apples, bananas, and dates through a Champion Juicer using the solid plate. In a large bowl, mix dough with vanilla, cinnamon, raisins, and walnuts. Spoon dough on a dehydrator tray with a teflex sheet and form into small round cookies. Dehydrate at 105° for 4 – 6 hours, turn cookies over and remove teflex sheet. Continue dehydrating for 4 – 6 hours or until desired moisture is obtained.

Seed Sauce

This sauce is wonderful over sliced fruit. The seeds are high in protein and calcium. For those with blood sugar concerns, the seeds slow the release of glucose from the fruit and create a more gradual release into the system. The result is a stabilization of blood sugar and a satiation of hunger for longer periods of time. By reducing the water, you can achieve the consistency of pudding and serve as a baby food or pie filling.

½ cup sunflower seeds that have been soaked at least
   4 hours and drained.
2 T water (more or less for desired consistency)
1 ripe banana

Optional: Add chopped dates, raisins, cinnamon, or substitute almonds for the seeds.

Blend all in a blender and serve immediately. The above quantities serve one.

Bibliography

Cousens, Gabriel, M.D. *Conscious Eating.* Essene Vision Books, 1997.

Diamond, Harvey and Marilyn. *Fit for Life.* Warner Books, 1985.

Diamond, Marilyn. *The American Vegetarian Cookbook.* Warner Books, 1990

McDougall, John, M.D. *The McDougall Program.* Penguin Books, 1990.

Szekely, Edmond Bordeaux. *The Essene Way, Biogenic Living.* Intl. Biogenic Society, 1981.

Wolfe, David. *The Sunfood Diet Success System.* Maul Brothers Publishing, 1999.

Yntema, Sharon K. *Vegetarian Children.* McBooks Press, 1987.

Raw and Living Food Resources

Books:

Conscious Eating by Gabriel Cousens, M.D. Essene Vision Books.

God's Way to Ultimate Health by Dr. George H. Malkmus. Hallelujah Acres Publishing.

Nature's First Law: The Raw-Food Diet, by Arlin, Dini, Wolfe. Maul Bros. Publishing.

Spiritual Nutrition and the Rainbow Diet by Gabriel Cousens, M.D. Cassandra Books.

Superior Nutrition by Herbert Shelton. Willow Publishing, Inc.

Survival into the 21st Century by Viktoras Kulvinskas, M.S. 21st Century Publications.

The Sunfood Diet Success System by David Wolfe. Maul Bros. Publishing

The Sprouting Book by Ann Wigmore. Avery Publishing Group

Raw-Food Recipe Books:

Dining in the Raw by Rita Romano. Kensington Books

Raw-Food Recipe Books – continued:

Living in the Raw, Recipes for a Healthy Lifestyle by Rose Lee Calabro. Rose Publishing.

The Garden of Eden Raw Fruit & Vegetable Recipes by Phyllis Avery. Hygeia Publishing.

The Raw Gourmet by Nomi Shannon. Alive Books.

The UnCook Book by Elizabeth Baker. ProMotion Publishing.

Organizations:

Nature's First Law
P. O. Box 900202
San Diego CA 92190
619-596-7979
(800) 205-2350 – orders
Web Site: http//www.rawfood.com
Email: nature@rawfood.com

Extensive catalog of everything to do with raw food. Virtually every raw food book in print. Juicers, dehydrators, videos and audio tapes and raw food items.

Hallelujah Acres
P. O. Box 2388
Shelby, NC 28151
(704) 481-1700

Hallelujah Acres was founded by Rev. George Malkmus. They provide publications, lectures and Health Ministries, advocating an 80% raw-food vegetarian diet.

Healthful Living International
P. O. Box 256
Sebatopol, CA 95473
(707) 887-9132
Email: info@healthfullivingintl.com
Web Site: http://www.healthfullivingintl.com
A pro-raw food organization led by Healthful Living Consultants who guide people to health via edication, counseling, fasting and healthful lifestyle.

Fresh Network
P. O. Box 71
Ely, Cambs, CB7 4GU, United Kingdom
Phone +44 (0) 870-800-7070
Email: info@fresh-network.com
Web Site: www.fresh-network.com
Fresh Network is an international network to exchange information, ideas and personal experiences so that individuals can change their diet and life-style with help and support from others, to suit their own personal set of ever changing needs and circumstances.

Periodicals:

Living Nutrition Magazine
64 pages - Contact is Dave Klein, (707) 887-9132
Email: dave@livingnutrition.com
Web Site: www.livingnutrition.com

Get Fresh! The official magazine of the Fresh Network
(4 issues per year)
P. O. Box 71

Ely, Cambs, CB7 4GU, United Kingdom
Phone: +44 (0) 870-800-7070
Email: info@fresh-network.com
Web Site: www.fresh-network.com

Internet Sources:

Nature's First Law:
http://www.rawfood.com

Raw Food Online Community:
http://www.living-foods.com

Living Nutrition Magazine:
http://www.livingnutrition.com

Fresh Network:
http://www.fresh-network.com

Mail Order Sources for Raw Food Items:

Date People
P. O. Box 808
Niland CA 92257
(760) 359-3211
Email: datefolk@brawleyonline.com

The Date People carry over 50 varieties of organic dates. The dates are raw, organic and non–hydrated. They offer reasonable prices and fast service.

Nature's Path Foods, Inc.
2220 Nature's Path Way
Blaine WA 98230

Email: response@naturespath.net
Web Site: naturespath.com

Nature's Path Foods is the maker of manna bread, sometimes called Essene Bread. The bread is available through most natural food stores.

Sun Organic Farms
P. O. Box 2429
Valley Center CA 92082
(888) 269-9888
Web Site: www.sunorganic.com

Sun Organic Farm carries raw, organic nuts, seeds, sprouting beans and grains, sun–ripened olives, dried fruit and vegetables, herbs and spices and sprouting equipment at very reasonable prices.

The Sprout House
17267 Sundance Dr.
Ramona, CA 92065
(800) 777-6887
Email: info@SproutHouse.com
Web Site: www.sprouthouse.com

The Sprout House carries many varieties of organic sprouting seeds and sprouting equipment.

Nature's First Law
P. O. Box 900202
San Diego, CA 92190
(800) 205-2350 or (619) 596-7979
Email: nature@rawfood.com - Web Site: www.rawfood.com

About the Author

Solomae (previously known as Cheryl Stoycoff) is a contemporary Christian Mystic, spiritual teacher, author and ordained minister who has experienced both the Eastern and Western spiritual paradigms and now assists others who seek to follow the true path of Christ. She draws upon her experiences of advanced states of consciousness, including the Christing process, to assist others in navigating the perils, pitfalls and complexities of moving into higher spiritual awareness.

Solomae has now retired from public appearances. Much of her time is now spent focusing on planetary healing and clearing. She is the author of five books and numerous recordings.

Solomae and her husband, Clyde Stoycoff, enjoy a quiet life in northeastern Oklahoma with their two sons, Zack and Kyle.

Living Spirit Foundation

Living Spirit Foundation and the Church of the Living Spirit is a non-profit 501(c)(3) spiritual organization and church. We are a Christ-centered, non-denominational and inner-faith ministry.

The purpose of the Living Spirit Ministry is to provide a means by which people can feel comfortable exploring their spirituality and moving beyond the confines of organized religion into the direct experience of God. We seek to unite through the transcendence of religious differences and a return to the pure message of the Christ, before Christianity molded it to fit the world. We seek to assist others in discovering the Christ directly within themselves and in manifesting it externally for the healing of humanity. We believe in the oneness of all, the power of love to transcend all differences, and the spiritual body within mankind as a real and tangible power for transformation.

We provide programs and services to assist others in developing their spiritual gifts in the ministry of Divine service, self-awareness and spiritual growth. Our programs include a Ministerial Ordination Program, On-line Courses, published materials and an extensive website providing free information on various aspects of the spiritual journey.

To Contact Us:

Living Spirit Foundation

P. O. Box 924

Claremore, OK 74018

Phone: (918) 341-1152

Email: info@livingspiritfoundation.org

Web Site: www.livingspiritfoundation.org